My Mother,
Munchausen's
and Me

My Mother, Munchausen's and Me

Helen Naylor

Thread

Published by Thread in 2021

An imprint of Storyfire Ltd.
Carmelite House
50 Victoria Embankment
London EC4Y 0DZ

www.thread-books.com

ISBN: 978-1-90977-068-3
eBook ISBN: 978-1-80019-799-2

Printed and bound in Great Britain

The FSC® label means that materials used for the product
have been responsibly sourced.

Prologue

There was a time when I loved my mother.

It's shocking – unnatural – to imply that I stopped loving my mum. But nothing about our relationship was normal.

Mum used to be everything I admired, the epitome of what a woman should be. In my eyes she was beautiful, good and perfect and we were tied together tightly. When I was older, my friends would mock me – 'You talk to her every day?' – as if we were too close, as if it was weird. But I'd been her carer throughout my childhood; we were symbiotically tied through her disabilities.

Society takes it for granted that mothers are good. They're supposed to love and care and have natural maternal instincts that make them compassionate and benevolent. Any bad behaviour can be dismissed as misguided affection, because mothers always love their children and always do their best for them. Mothers are good.

My mother wasn't good.

She presented herself as a loving parent, a genuine friend and a vulnerable victim, but that wasn't the truth. My mother faked debilitating illnesses for thirty years and her pretence of disability moulded my family and stole my childhood. Her manipulations forced me to sacrifice and compromise because she appeared to be unwell, and I did it because I loved her. Everything I knew about myself – my identity and my upbringing – relied on the belief that I was the daughter of two physically disabled parents. Except that was a lie.

The mother I thought I had was an illusion. I didn't know the real her at all, and it's impossible to love a ghost. But though I no longer love Mum, I don't hate her. It isn't indifference either. Rather she's trapped in a vacuum inside of me, unable to be categorised, frozen in my numb mind. I still miss her. Not the real her of course; I miss the mum I thought I had, the one who loved me.

Even my thoughts and memories are skewed by Mum's version of the truth. Take my first memory. I'm sitting on the stairs in my parents' house, aged three, with my best friend, Carys. It was summer and the staircase was the coolest place we could find, so we sat at the top where it curved onto the landing, leaning against the wall in our shorts and tees to eat some sweets that had melted into the wax paper. We spent an age trying to peel the gluey sweets away, our fingers covered in sticky, unsatisfying gloop, until we gave up and started eating them whole, wrapper and all. It's a happy, funny, wholesome memory.

The problem is, this happened almost a year after my *real* first memory. I remember standing on a chair at my friend's house pretending to decorate the wall with a large, blue children's paint brush. I remember falling off, landing on my arm and being taken to hospital. This memory is a much darker story of a little girl broken and abused at the hands of her most trusted parent. I believed it happened when I was four because Mum told me it happened much later than it really did. She manipulated it in time and in its retelling so I didn't understand what had really occurred. Like everything else in her life, it was a carefully whittled lie.

If it weren't for the diaries, I might never have known the truth about this memory or anything else that happened in my childhood. Every day for fifty-five years my mum wrote about her daily life, from when she was twelve in the 1960s to a year before her death. For someone else, reading their parent's diary entries might be a tearful delight. For a historian they're a wonderful social history. But for me they're something else. Reading them, I was able to do a psychological autopsy and discover who the ghost really was. And, as I unravelled my mother, I unravelled myself.

Chapter One

Photograph

Even after thirty years I can clearly recall my maternal grandparents' house, the black and white semi cemented into my memory as strongly as my own childhood home. Nanny and Grampy's house had a stern black lacquered door that opened onto a busy street. I can still feel the luxuriously deep carpet beneath my feet, my toes sinking into the soft, caramel fluff, and see Nanny in her pink slippers standing in the kitchen doorway with an apron tied around her middle. She had a warm, wide waist to snuggle into and she used to sneak me perfectly snapped pieces of chocolate. On the cupboard behind her in the kitchen there was a poster of a pig which provoked hilarity, but I couldn't read so didn't get the joke.

Grampy's garden was full of tomatoes and prized marrows and was overlooked by a train track that provided a reassuring background noise as engines whizzed past. Grampy was the tallest person I knew, always smartly dressed. Most vividly I remember sitting on his lap. He'd complain his leg was itching but would tickle my knee instead.

Sometimes Mum told me stories of her childhood, like the legend of when the flood came. She told me that the rain fell and covered the roads until canoes were the only transport. The water rose up, filling the house and pushing my grandparents, my mum and my aunt upstairs to escape. What was it Grampy went back to get? Whatever it was, he didn't reach it; he was trapped by the flood, clinging on in the kitchen for dear life, the rushing water trying to sweep him away. It was my aunt who was the hero: a plucky teen who entered the water and dragged him through the waist-deep, sewage-filled torrent and up the stairs to safety. The four of them watched the water rise until it almost reached the landing, fretting how they'd get onto the roof. But it slowly ebbed away, dropping back down the steps, revealing the mess left behind. Mum told me that this was how she and Dad began to court, after he helped her family get back to normal.

I enjoyed being with my grandparents and yet, at the same time, there was a loneliness to it. The curse of not having siblings is to be a child in an adult's world. I would often creep upstairs, the grown-ups' voices a low drone emanating from the living room below as I trespassed into the bedrooms. My favourite was the small front room hung with glittering, blue-green wallpaper, like peacocks' feathers, covered in iridescent fairies. I would watch these tiny, winged characters closely, willing them to pop out of the paper and play.

I remember pausing on the landing on one of these occasions and seeing, for the first time, a framed picture balanced precariously on the banister. It was a slightly faded photograph of the family from before I was born; my grandparents stood in the middle with my aunt to one side and my parents on the other. My dad, Alan, was the shortest one among them at only five foot five, my mum towering above him. He looked remarkably similar to Ian Hislop, but with glasses. His rounded face was emphasised by his sagging jowls and a large belly as he aged, but in the photo he was young and fit with a soft wave of light brown hair and a big, broad smile – a rare show of happiness.

My mum, Elinor, was almost as tall as Grampy and she stood out in the family for being so slim. Even back then she reminded me of Margaret Thatcher: the same pointed nose, permed hair and small slits for eyes, though Mum's were hidden behind gold-rimmed spectacles. Unlike Thatcher, she never wore power suits or heels. She was the queen of polyester, her dresses chosen from the classic section of Marks and Spencer. Her shoulders were slumped and resigned, her driver shoes flat and rounded. Dad's arm was around her in the photo and she was smiling too.

I studied the photo and thought how complete the family looked without me. I didn't fit in. I wondered if I'd been adopted. It was a big thought for a small girl. It was undeniable that I was my parents' daughter since I shared their features and their piercing, blue eyes, but I felt an otherness about me – even at four – of being an unwanted outsider in the intimacy of my little family. And yet I can't remember why I felt like that, only that I was already unhappy.

Chapter Two

Mothballs

My home town had a prestigious past full of stories of castles, medieval kings and Civil War strongholds, but by the time I was born in the 1980s, it had settled into a small, self-sufficient rural town in the Midlands. Redundant of good transport links it was a haven for independent shops and mediocre facilities, having neither enough in the locality to compel its teenage citizens to look beyond, nor to prevent their dissatisfaction. It was a beautiful, but isolated, backwater.

Our house sat on the main road into town, the yellow-cream render jarring against the other neat, white semis. Once, so Mum and Dad said, they'd had a life beyond our house. They would cycle to work at the bank and go sailing at weekends. But none of that was familiar to me because it had ended when I was seven. Both my parents had become disabled that year, coinciding with their redundancies from work.

Although I knew Dad was more seriously ill with heart and lung problems, it was Mum's disabilities that ruled our lives. Dad might have emphysema, but it was self-inflicted by forty years of smoking and later, when he was diagnosed with cardiomyopathy, it was dismissed by Mum as an inherited problem that lacked status. But Mum's ME or chronic fatigue syndrome was mysterious and uncertain. It had differing origin myths, the most common explanation being that, because of me, she'd overdone it when she'd had the flu. Sometimes she would say it had been triggered by using mothballs in her wardrobe, or that it was a leftover effect from her undiagnosed postnatal depression, but these alternative stories were only brought out when she was in company far away from the friends who knew her well. Mum was enthralled with the ME, spending all her time researching it, talking about it and going to the ME group. I knew it was her favourite child.

Mum had stopped cooking and cleaning since her diagnosis, and she couldn't walk me to school or even down to the corner shop. Her need for rests in the afternoons meant no day trips out and there were few visitors.

Since my grandparents had died, there was a new story about my closest relations. Mum had told me before that Nanny and Grampy had been born into mining families in Wales but, by fortunate serendipity, Grampy had been plucked out of this dusty, dirty poverty by a Dickensian-style benefactor and enrolled into a private school. He became the family prodigy working in, and later owning, a pharmacy. It was storybook rags to riches.

Now Mum added a darker streak to this story. Nanny was a hypochondriac, prone to fears about her health after an operation on her thyroid went wrong and left her with lifelong complications. Grampy was a workaholic, either at his pharmacy or building social connections, mainly absent from the family's life. There were constant marital arguments, with my grandparents shouting and screaming while my mother cowered upstairs. And my aunt was the favourite, constantly pandered to by her parents, leaving her free to bully her demure older sister. It had been a difficult, damaging childhood for Mum.

After my grandparents' deaths, we'd become estranged from my aunt. Mum said she'd been forced to break contact with her sister to protect us. She painted my aunt as a terrifyingly dangerous person, though no details were given to me about this and, being a child, I simply took Mum's word for it.

Even the family friends and relations we still had contact with were kept at a distance and their annual visits were the only invasion into our otherwise isolated lives. At the time I didn't understand that it wasn't normal to have to describe who you were to your family when you called at Christmas, to find yourself running out of ways to identify yourself before they realised who you were.

The three of us had fallen into a familiar routine. After lunch each day, Dad would go to the pub, Mum would go to bed for a rest and I was left to fill every afternoon of every weekend and holiday for the rest of my childhood. It wasn't until I was a parent myself that I realised that this wasn't normal behaviour. Until then I wouldn't have questioned why my parents would leave a primary-aged child without supervision, without anything to entertain me, without any thought to my safety. I wouldn't have thought to call it neglect.

I remember lying on the sofa one day, listening to the stillness, the heat of the summer afternoon making the room humid and stifling. I'd played in the garden for a while, dancing as I did loops of the perimeter, softly singing tunes that played in my head. And when the day had become too hot, I'd gone inside and found some scrap paper and written a story about a ten-year-old girl like me, who climbed into the loft and disappeared into a different world. Sometimes I might get out my board games – played once with my parents and then put away in a cupboard – and make up my own rules so I could play them alone. But on that particular day I stared vacantly at the TV screen, the sound down so low that I had to lip read, hopelessly wishing there was something on that I wanted to watch.

Time ceased to exist here, in the vacuum of my afternoons. It was one long emptiness, a desert land where I longed for Dad to come home or Mum to get up, or someone – anyone – to take me out into the sunshine. There had been a couple of thirst-quenching afternoons when Dad didn't go to the pub, instead taking me to the garden centre to look at the pets. We'd had a drink in the sun-drenched conservatory – him a coffee and me a Coke – and both times he'd bought me a book. There was a lot of quiet between us, but it was like an oasis in the desert of my loneliness.

Most days, however, were like this one: silent and solitary. Even when we went on holiday, it was the same and, while Mum rested in our room and Dad sat in the bar, I'd wander corridors or stare at the unreachable sea sparkling in the sunshine through the windows of the hotel lobby.

I dragged myself up from the sofa and opened the living room door just enough so I could squeeze through without it squeaking. The hallway was cold, the rectangle of patterned glass reflecting a creepy Chinese dragon across the green, paisley carpet. In the winter, when the house became dark much earlier, I would wait there to see if the monster would leap out at me. It was easier not to be afraid in the summer, when the house was sunny all afternoon: much better than when I had to fumble in the darkness, not wanting to waste electricity by putting the lights on.

I knew exactly how to climb the stairs so I was soundless, the pattern well established in my muscle memory. Miss the first two, keep to the right, jump the sixth step, side-step to the left. I didn't falter – left, right, left, middle – to avoid the ones that creaked. I paused at the top and waited, my ears straining to hear for Mum stirring in bed. The silence equalled success and I'd come to pride myself on my ninja abilities.

I went into my room, holding the handle down until the door was closed, the slow release meaning it clicked quietly. Sitting on my bed, I stared out at the gardens beyond my window, the large oak tree on the opposite street, green and full, hiding the road beyond. It was my familiar, reliable companion, and soon it would shift gently, its leaves reddening and falling until the sparse winter branches made shadows on my wall in the car lights.

I opened my cupboard and took out my dolls, laid them on the floor and played, their imaginary voices speaking only in my head.

The clock showed there was at least another hour of muted restraint ahead of me, but I was used to it now. I could even cry in silence. I was doing so well at hiding myself that I thought soon I might become completely invisible.

Chapter Three

Washing Machine

Carys was an intrepid adventurer, an explorer of possibilities and new creations. With wild, onyx hair; piercing, dark eyes and a freedom I'd never had, she was everything I wanted to be. She'd been my best friend since I was tiny and now, aged ten, we knew each other so well that our thoughts were entwined. When I wasn't on my own, I was with Carys, our afternoons at my house entirely unsupervised.

Den building felt like a vocation. We were survival experts in the jungle, problem solvers in space, architects of our imaginations. Usually we built them in bedrooms, but Mum needed quiet for her rest, so that day we built our den in the hall space. The downstairs rooms of my parents' house ran in an interconnecting circle and we'd engineered our den between the stairs and one of the doors to the kitchen, pinning sheets with pegs and lining the floor with pillows. It had been a logistically difficult job, one of the toughest challenges we'd faced in our den career, but we'd finally got it secure. Scrunched up in our makeshift tent, we huddled together conspiratorially, eating sweets.

'How did this conversation start?' I said.

'The cats… next door… my grandparents…'

'Next weekend!' I said, pulling a duvet up around me.

'Oh yeah. My cousins.'

'Haven't seen them in ages.'

'Nah, they've been—'

The firm, loud thud stopped Carys's words in her mouth. We eyeballed each other, our ears straining. It was the sound of the back door being kicked. It was the sound of someone breaking into the kitchen. For a moment we didn't move, not daring to make a noise. When Carys spoke again, her voice caught in her throat.

'What was that?'

'Shhh!' I hissed. 'It's a burglar.'

Carys set her brown eyes on me, thoroughly unconvinced. But the next clunk made her jump.

'What do we do?' she said, her voice dropping to copy mine.

'Get something we can hit them with,' I whispered. 'A baseball bat.'

'A baseball bat?' she said, shrugging her shoulders.

'Alright, an umbrella.'

We tiptoed into the lounge, leaning around the door to check where the intruders were, my heart pounding and stopping me from seeing straight. I slunk towards the kitchen, the umbrella gripped tightly in my hands. With every footstep my belief that we could defeat and outwit any adult dribbled away, but I knew I couldn't disturb Mum. It didn't even cross my mind to get her. As we entered the empty kitchen, I dropped my umbrella to my side.

'There's no one here.'

Carys was still holding her umbrella high in her hands and was glued to the corner of the room. I scanned blankly around the tiny box of a kitchen.

'The washing machine!' She pointed to the plumes of smoke rising.

'Mum!' I shouted, dropping the umbrella, but there was no response. 'Mum!' I shouted louder, running through the lounge and hammering up the stairs. 'Mum!'

When I got to her room, she was sitting in bed reading a magazine, her permed hair tousled in her usual post-nap look, her clothes crumpled. She gave me a withering look while I panted, as if I were bothering her with a silly game.

'The washing machine's on fire! There's smoke and it's making a funny noise…'

'Turn it off!' she yelled. 'Turn it off!'

I spun around as Mum pulled back the bedcovers and I ran back down the stairs shouting to Carys. It didn't strike me as strange then, Mum telling a child – and not even her own child – to stay in the room and touch the sparking electrical appliance. It was normal for me to feel responsible for her.

I burst into the kitchen and ran to Carys's side. We searched for the right button on the wobbling, white box as the room continued to fill with smoke, running our fingers across the cryptic signs on the control panel. Neither of us had ever used a washing machine and neither of us knew what to do.

There was an explosion as Mum struggled through the kitchen door. She hadn't followed me through the living room, instead ploughing through our den leaving pegs and sheets everywhere.

'Not there. The plug on the wall!' she shouted, pushing us out of the way.

The washing machine fell still as soon as she clicked it off, an act too simple for such a dramatic moment. The smell of burning was stinging my eyes.

'Alright then,' Mum said, spinning sharply towards us and shooing us. 'You can go off and play.'

The adrenaline was throbbing in my veins making me want to laugh and cry simultaneously.

'We thought it was a burglar,' I said, the acrid smoke catching in my throat.

Mum batted me away.

We dragged the umbrellas back into the hall and stood staring at the damage to our den. It was completely destroyed, a mere pile of parts that no longer made up the small, safe snug we'd built. I stared at it unable to pull my eyes away, my mind whirring. What would have happened if someone had been breaking in? Mum hadn't come when I called – not the first time, nor the second time, nor the third.

We were in the living room when Carys's mum came to pick her up. Petite and very Welsh, Carys's mum, Lynn, was like an auntie to me. She had a warm manner and was tremendous fun, a very different creature to my mum, yet they were good friends. Carys and I used to joke that we could leave our mothers together for a week and they'd still be chatting. We'd long since learnt that 'We're going in a minute' was meaningless.

'I've learnt to draw Danger Mouse,' Carys said as we stood waiting, hands dug into our jean pockets.

'No way,' I said. 'Show me?'

I slipped between our mums as they stood at the edge of the sofa and searched through the piles of stationery hidden in the darkness behind the settee. I rifled through boxes of pens, the distant drone of the conversation drifting over my head, like a radio buzz in the background.

'The doctor said it's very serious,' Mum said, and my ears pricked, my fingers slowing as I foraged. 'Alan's mother probably had the same thing and she died very young, very suddenly.'

I knew that story. I knew that, long before I was born, my paternal grandmother had called the doctor for my sick grandfather and, as she opened the door, she'd fallen down dead on the carpet. There was no explanation, no build up, but I'd understood that sometimes that's what happens. People just die.

'Apparently,' Mum said, her voice trilling, 'he could drop dead at any moment.'

I stood up slowly, my pulse racing, and Mum met me with a twinkling grin. There was a moment as our eyes connected – my heart utterly motionless – when I knew that she was thrilled I'd overheard.

'What?' she said, shrugging slightly.

I waited, expecting something more, but she only shrugged again to dismiss me. I sank back down into the shadows, my heart pounding. The doctor had said Dad could drop dead at any moment. My dad who did all the jobs around the house, who cared for Mum, who kept everything going. If Dad died – or was it when Dad died? – I would have to replace him as Mum's carer because there was no one else to help us. I knew, instinctively, that I'd have to give up all my dreams of leaving home and going to university. All the responsibility would be on me. Maybe I'd even have to leave school to care for her.

'Have you found it?' Carys said, hunkering down beside me.

'Oh, yeah,' I said, passing her the paper and pens. 'Yeah, let's see.'

I pretended to pay attention as Carys drew a perfect cartoon replica, my head ablaze with panic. The plans were already falling into place to ensure that I was ready when Dad dropped dead. It could be any time, any day. I felt the burden entirely on me, the responsibility for my parents on my small shoulders alone. I had to be ready to take control because if I wasn't, then no one would be holding the wheel. It was only a brief moment, one that I was supposed to forget. But it changed me forever. From that day, aged ten, I knew that the responsibility for my mother lay entirely on me.

Elinor's Diary

1st August 1993
Carys over, played while I rested and Alan went out, the washing machine burnt out and Helen and Carys braved the smoke. Alan came home but everything ok. He broke open machine to get washing out – done.

Chapter Four

Christmas Drinks

'Here they are,' Mum announced, jumping up from the sofa to rush to the door.

The Christmas tree was up in the window, decorated in a gaudy mix of ancient and modern ornaments in every colour and material. It reflected my parents' equally eclectic lounge: a combination of styles of furniture, a crazy-paving fireplace and textured cream wallpaper. Mum had prepared nibbles, Dad had arranged the bottles in the cocktail cabinet and we were all dressed up for the visitors. Mum was wearing a burgundy dress with a laced collar and shoulder pads, Dad a slightly nicer than usual shirt and slacks, and me checked trousers and a matching hat that I bought from Tammy Girl. I felt very grown up, definitely more like fourteen than twelve.

'Happy birthday.'

'Thank you,' Judy said, taking off her coat and passing it to Mum. 'Wow, you've grown again, Helen.'

'Hello, Judy,' Dad said. 'Haven't seen you since…'

'This time last year.'

'What can I get you to drink?'

I sat in the chair by the window – the one that was only ever used on Christmas Eve – self-consciously crossing my legs and admiring my new trousers. I liked these special evenings with Judy and Paul, two of the many 'aunts' and 'uncles' who lived on the periphery of my life, whom I adored completely because I saw so little of them. We rarely saw any family members any more, not since my grandparents died and Mum had become estranged from her sister because – Mum said – of my aunt's bullying behaviour. Contact was limited with the relatives we did still see and our irregular visits a couple of times a year were all I knew of most of my family. Similarly, when I was a child, our family friends were distant, kept to a few annual get togethers. Mum's closest relationships were carefully managed, mainly carried out on the phone; long, nightly conversations where she had total control of the narrative. I was stranded in her truth without any other adults to intervene. Dad and I weren't close, by his choice or perhaps by Mum's, and there were no other grown-ups, friends or relatives who saw more than Mum's version of events. Without anyone to contradict, her perspective was my truth entirely.

Before they retired, my parents had worked with Judy at the bank. Situated in the centre of town, the looming, grey structure with cathedral doors contained a labyrinth of narrow corridors, punctuated by pockets where my parents' friends worked behind glass dividers. The bank was a place of legends; it was where my parents had met. Mum told me that she hadn't liked Dad at first, but that after the flood she'd fallen for him.

'I was given three options when I left school,' Mum had told me while we sat on her bed one day after school. 'Teaching, nursing or secretarial work. I said I didn't want to do any of those. And do you know what they said?'

I'd shaken my head, enthralled.

'The careers advisor told me that they couldn't help me. But I got a job in the bank, took night classes, worked damn hard. I was the only woman to pass the exams and I was better than all the men I worked with. Everyone said I could have flown up the promotion ladder. But my manager told me he'd never advance me instead of a man.'

'No!' I'd gasped, sitting up straighter in the bed, feeling outraged.

'Oh yes!' she'd said, her pleasure in retelling the story like a warm haze around her. 'Of course, that was the seventies. I had to sit in that job while the moronic men that I was training went on to greater things. I could have done their work in my sleep, but they wouldn't promote a woman.'

By the time I was twelve Judy was rising the ranks and would soon make manager, and it went unsaid that Mum could have been in the same position if she hadn't left the bank to have me. I simultaneously held the conflicting beliefs that Mum considered my birth to have ruined her life by stealing her from the bank while also knowing she wasn't jealous of Judy's career. I knew from Mum's subtle comments that she believed she was superior to her friend: little snipes about how quickly she could count money, how incapable she considered many of her former colleagues, how exceptional she had been at her job. I swallowed everything she said to me without question, no matter how contradictory it was.

'No one expected me to have a baby, not then. I was thirty-five – that was old to start having children in the eighties,' she'd said, although the story was well worn. 'But I said to your dad that it was our last chance, and we had a big talk. In the end your dad said, "We'll try, and if we get pregnant, then that's fine. But if not, then it doesn't matter".'

The story of my conception hung over me like a sign above my head. Mum had smiled and chuckled and I'd copied her because I found their lack of broodiness funny too. But when we stopped laughing, it ached in my chest.

'I went back to work after you were born,' Mum had continued. 'But when redundancies came along, my role was one of the first to go. Still, it took three men to do my job.'

Judy was the same age as Mum, but she drove a fast car and had a fashionable haircut, trendy clothes and bright make-up: a stark contrast to Mum's calf-length floral skirts and dowdy blouses, her penchant for beige and peach.

'Is this new, this record player?' Paul asked.

'Yes,' Dad said. 'We can put our music onto tapes now.'

'Tapes are all the rage now,' Paul said. 'I went to Richards' Music Store the other day. The record players come with all sorts of fancy things now, nothing I want, so I said, "I want a normal one," and the owner said, "We don't do that sort of thing any more, you're out of date," and I said, "I don't think money ever goes out of date though does it? You find me one."'

I covered my mouth with my hand. Even when the details of Paul's stories went over my head, I enjoyed listening to the calm tide of his voice.

'I did some wrangling,' Paul continued, sharing a wink with Judy, who smirked at Mum, 'and in the end he offered it for ten quid as long as I didn't come back.'

'Isn't he terrible?' Judy laughed, an inviting giggle that drew us in. 'Did you hear Brian retired finally?'

'I never thought he would.'

'He should have gone years ago.'

'Alan! Did you hear that?'

'What's that?' Dad said, arriving from the kitchen with drinks.

'Brian's retired.'

'About time.'

'That's what Judy said.'

I sat close-mouthed, letting the adult conversation drain over me, feeling like a fly on the wall, unseen and unheard.

'And how are you, Helen?' Judy said, turning to me.

I coughed a little at using my voice. 'I'm okay.'

'How's school?'

'Good, thanks.'

Mum tutted. 'She's doing really good. She's in the top sets, got a glowing report.'

'That's great.'

'Especially bearing in mind my ME being so bad. But I make sure it doesn't impact Helen at all.'

'Is it no better then?'

I leant on my hand and looked at the clock. Judy and Paul had arrived less than half an hour before, but this signalled the turn in the evening. Every year it was the same thing, the fun bit would end, and Mum would dominate the conversation for the next few hours. I knew I could let my attention wander, curl up my legs on the comfy chair and then, in a short while, I could make my excuses and go upstairs.

'No, not at all better. I have to sleep for eighteen hours a day.'

'Eighteen hours?'

'It's crippling, absolutely crippling.'

In my head I counted how long Mum was in bed each day. No matter how I tried to skew the figures, it didn't add up to eighteen. And anyway, Mum didn't sleep, she read magazines or watched TV. *Whatever*, I told myself, *she spends a lot of time in bed, even if she is exaggerating*.

Judy nodded but Paul was screwing his face up. Dad had gone back to the kitchen to make more drinks and Mum was monologuing, seated like a queen on her throne, addressing her audience who were beginning to slump in their seats. But it was no matter to Mum; this was her favourite subject, and she wouldn't be put off. I crept out of the room, and no one looked round. My invisibility was complete.

Chapter Five

Mirror

'I've put that mirror on top on my wardrobe, do you see?'

We lay on Mum's bed, the heat of the summer sun burning through the shiny peach curtains, making me feel nauseous. I'd got bored a while ago, having exhausted all afternoon entertainment options, and peeked around Mum's door to find her watching TV.

Before Mum cut contact with my aunt, she was the one I'd chat to like this. She'd taught me about periods and make-up, she'd listened to my pre-teen questions and indulged my musical tastes. But at fourteen, now I was no longer allowed to see my aunt, Mum was the only adult who spent time talking and listening to me.

'I can see who comes to the front door and then I know whether to get up.'

'And if it's someone you don't want to see, then you can stay in bed?'

'Exactly,' she laughed, smoothing her patterned cream skirt. 'You've always understood.'

I turned over and gazed up at her. Side on I could see the red impression her glasses had left on the bridge of her large nose, the untouched curls next to her face and the flattened hair at the back.

'When I first got ME,' she said, looking down at me, 'no one believed me. Not my parents, not my friends – not even your dad.'

'Really?'

'Good friends of mine – like Annette – she was really cynical, said it was all in my mind. Even your dad thought I was making it up. You were only seven, but you believed me.'

She lay back a moment and closed her eyes, an antiques programme humming in the background. 'We have a very special relationship. It's not at all like I was with my mother.'

'Really?' I said, 'In what way?'

She sighed thoughtfully. 'My mother and I were very different. But we've always been the same, you and me. That's why we're so close.'

I laid back on the pillows feeling dozy and satisfied, keeping a soft focus on the TV for a moment before my attention wandered. Our equally pale legs were laid side by side, my denim shorts revealing more skin than Mum's mid-length skirt, our calves and ankles the same thinly curved shape.

'Your legs are so long.'

'Yes,' Mum said, matter-of-fact, pulling her skirt up a little. 'It's what attracted your dad to me. My beautiful legs. Back in the seventies it was all miniskirts, and he couldn't keep his eyes off me.'

I turned to my own shorter version.

'You should have been taller,' she said, as if reading my mind. 'You were supposed to be as tall as me, but I don't know what went wrong. You've got tiny feet and hands too. Not like mine.'

She extended her arm as if to prove it, examining her long, slender fingers, perfectly manicured nails, delicate English rose skin. Everything about her was perfect.

'Piano player fingers, if only I'd have learnt.' She took my hand in hers and examined it. 'You'd have better hands if you stopped biting your nails. But your fingers are stumpy anyway.'

She let my hand fall, taking up a china cup and saucer patterned with strawberries and rimmed in gold from her bedside table.

'The thing is,' she said, taking a sip. 'I'm the same shape as my dad. Tall, slim and slight. And you're the same shape as your dad.'

'Oh, you're hiding up here,' said Dad, as if on cue. 'I've been trying to find you.'

He was out of breath from climbing the stairs, his plaid shirt tight across his bulging beer belly, bloated by steroids. His health had declined in the previous few years, though in my memory he had always looked like this: short and fat and wheezing.

I looked down at my stubby fingers, my stunted legs, my waist. My body was such a disappointment, a hopeful possibility fallen short. Short and Fat and Ugly.

'We were talking about how my legs attracted you to me,' Mum said with a large smile. I could read every tiny inflection she made, and I knew she was mocking him.

'Oh, right,' he said, looking down at the floor. 'I'll leave you girls to chat then. More tea?'

'Yes please.'

I listened to Dad struggling downstairs, taking each step with cumbersome heaviness. I could picture him clinging onto the banister, pausing at the bottom to recover. He hated the heat. The humidity lay thickly on his chest and he struggled to breathe.

'Did I tell you?' Mum said, interrupting my thoughts. 'My cousin, Louise, had her baby? They've called it Elinor.'

I followed the pattern of the Artex ceiling, my hands and feet too weighty to move. I couldn't believe anyone would call their baby Elinor. It seemed so antiquated.

'How did you come up with my name?' I asked, hoping she didn't expect me to give an opinion on the baby's moniker. I'd long felt self-conscious of my name. I wanted to be a Zoe or a Katie instead of an old-fashioned Helen. It was outdated, another sign that I was the child of older parents, along with Mum's embarrassing clothes, her walking stick and her insistence on using mobility scooters when we went shopping in town.

'I liked Estella, but your dad said no.'

'Estella?' I said, wrinkling my nose. 'Like in *Great Expectations*?'

'That's the one.'

'But she's horrible,' I said, sitting up straighter and turning to her. 'She's selfish and mean and taunting.'

'Yes,' she said, staring straight at me. 'I suppose so.'

She glanced up at her mirror, letting the words hang in the air. The room felt hot and close.

'Well, thank goodness for Dad,' I said, leaning back again.

'He liked Melanie.'

'I can't imagine being called Melanie.'

'No, I didn't like it either. But we both liked Helen so Helen it was.'

The antiques expert murmured from the fifteen-inch TV that sat on the dark wooden blanket box at the end of Mum's bed. Her room was framed in matching dark wood wardrobes, each crammed with clothes and shoes, most of which had never been worn, and her large, matching dressing table was full of old, decaying make-up: dodgy 1980s lipsticks that burnt my mouth when I tried them on.

'Did I tell you that you were born the night Karen Carpenter died?' she said, taking a slurp of tea. 'That's where you got your musical talents from.'

'From Karen Carpenter?' I said, screwing up my face.

'Well, it's strange, isn't it?' she said, shrugging and returning the cup to its coaster. 'No one else in our family is musical. And she died the same time you were born.'

I winced. 'You're saying I'm the reincarnation of Karen Carpenter?'

'It would explain a lot.'

'Like what?' I laughed. She got out of bed and sat at her dressing table.

'Oh, I don't know.' Taking up her rounded brush, she began to tease the flattened hair at the back of her head. 'Like how you play the guitar.'

After being given a few pop tapes in my tweens, I'd fallen in love with music. I listened on repeat to my two 'NOW That's What I Call Music' albums on my Walkman in the car, singing along with equal delight to Take That, Shanice and Jimmy Nail, innocently belting out the lyrics to 'Ebeneezer Goode' and 'Ain't 2 Proud 2 Beg' until my dad told me I was too loud. In my early teens the Radio 1 DJs became my close companions during the lonely afternoons, and the lyrics of every top 40 song became permanently etched in my memory. Meanwhile, Mum said she didn't like music. To me, this was a staggering statement. I could accept she didn't like the Britpop I enjoyed at fourteen, but to dismiss the whole concept of music felt outrageous, as if she were rejecting love or breathing. The house was filled with Radio 4 or local talk radio, and any music emanating from my room – either from the radio, my CD collection or the guitar I'd taught myself to play – was greeted with disgust and derision from my parents. They'd even apologised for the 'noise' to our bemused neighbours.

I sat up, letting my legs hang over the edge of the bed, and tightened my lips into a sarcastic smile. 'Because the only way I could play the guitar is if I'm the reincarnation of Karen Carpenter?'

'It's not such a strange idea,' she said, examining herself in the three-piece mirror. 'When you were little, you said you could remember being someone else before you were born. You said you could show me the place where you'd been buried.'

'Yeah,' I murmured. 'I remember that.'

I recalled crouching behind the sofa, desperately trying to think who I once had been as Mum pressed me to give more details. I told her my former name and the place where I'd been buried, unsure whether I was making it up or remembering a past life. Bringing up the memory felt like revealing a dirty secret: something deeply unsettling.

'Well then,' she said, catching my eye in the reflection, 'If you were some Victorian woman, maybe you were Karen Carpenter too.'

Chapter Six

Insomnia

The doctor's surgery had once been a grand Georgian villa and some of the side rooms had the wonky floorboards and elaborate fireplaces to prove it. I sat beside Mum, an awkward, skinny fourteen-year-old, twisting my fingers and listening to the anxious tick of the clock, the footsteps of patients on the tiled floor, the low-level chatter of the receptionists.

Mum was at ease in the surgery, flicking through a magazine, her hair styled and make-up thickly applied. It was her second home, a place she and Dad visited so often that she walked down the corridors as if she owned them and spoke to the receptionists like old friends. Despite all her appointments here, there was little concrete diagnosis, and she'd tut sarcastically when the tests came back negative. 'Typical,' she'd say. Instead, she resorted to buying herbal medications by post, tens of silvery blue bottles that were labelled with long, unpronounceable names of vitamins, minerals and probiotics. She said if she found the right combination, she would cure her ME with this mixture of coloured pills and chalky powders. There was a whole cupboard in our kitchen devoted to her remedies, while Dad's prescribed medication was hidden away in the dining room. There was so much of it he had to have a pill box labelled for times of the day rather than days of the week, but it was relegated to the sideboard, out of sight.

As for me, I rarely came to the doctor's, even when I was unwell. Mum usually overlooked any symptoms I had, and I often resorted to self-medicating out of her sight. I remember my feet were covered with verrucas for years and, even when I asked her what to do, she dismissed them as 'nothing'. I tried everything I could think of, digging at my soles with scissors, slathering them in antiseptic, but nothing worked. Eventually I saw an advert on TV and unearthed some wart cream from the bottom of the large, metal medicine box kept on Mum's side of the bed. I was amazed that these painful, disgusting holes in my feet disappeared so simply. Why hadn't Mum told me it was that easy to fix? I hated the disfiguring acne too, believing that it was my fault for not washing enough, or with the right soap. I spent my teens feeling ugly and deformed, the huge boil-like spots rising on my face, neck and back, believing there was nothing I could do. It wasn't until I got engaged, years later, that Mum told me to get some antibiotics from the GP. Within a few months I had perfect, spotless skin but I ached inside. Why hadn't she told me before? All those years I'd felt repulsive when a short trip to the doctor would have solved the problem.

It hadn't been my idea to come to the doctor this time, but Mum said it was a real concern, and that meant it was serious. She said it wasn't normal. She said it needed sorting. Her uncharacteristic insistence was unnerving. I bit my nails and fidgeted, unable to get comfortable on the hard wooden chairs.

'Miss Page, room four, Doctor Hopkinson.'

We trudged up the uneven stairs, Mum grasping onto the banister, her stick clicking on each step. The first floor was brighter than downstairs, but, despite the high ceiling, the side room was poky and claustrophobic. Dr Hopkinson was an anomaly in the surgery. She was young, pretty and female. I took the second seat as Mum settled in beside the doctor.

'How can I help you?'

'Helen, tell Dr Hopkinson,' Mum said.

She folded her arms across her chest and flashed narrowed, menacing eyes at me. I knew it had been a mistake to come here, to believe I needed to be seen. I struggled to swallow, my throat tight. Mum turned back to the doctor before I could reply.

'She says she can't sleep,' she announced, leaning back on her chair, eyebrows arched.

My fingernails dugs into my palms. I'd regretted telling Mum I couldn't sleep as soon as the words had escaped my mouth, somehow knowing I'd end up here, feeling powerless and under suspicion.

'Do you wake up in the night?' the doctor asked.

'No,' I said, my voice catching. 'It just takes me ages to get to sleep. Hours.'

Mum shared a look with the doctor. I wished we hadn't come.

'Are you worried about anything in particular?'

'I don't think so. I just think about things,' I said, my words fading into a long, accusatory silence.

'Well, I can't give you any drugs to stop you thinking, Helen,' the doctor chuckled, turning back to Mum who mirrored her laughter. 'Apart from something like anti-psychotics, and you don't want to go on those at fourteen.'

'No, she doesn't!' agreed Mum, crossing her legs towards Dr Hopkinson, her peach skirt dangling around her calf.

My face was hot and red. I gave a half laugh, hoping I was in on the joke too, and shuffled my feet awkwardly. I had wasted the doctor's time. It was the trivial complaint of a silly teenager: nothing important, nothing concerning. Dr Hopkinson was already moving on, ushering us out of the room and readying herself for her next *real* patient.

Mum led the way down the stairs, her pace much quicker now, her stick held high in the air as she descended. Marching outside with Margaret Thatcher's authoritarian bluster, she let the door swing back into my face. I looked at the ground, trailing her as she dodged puddles. Dad was waiting in the disabled bay directly outside the surgery, the sound of his favourite talk radio humming. Mum slammed the door as she got into the front seat, and I felt the weight of her back to me. I willed the floor to swallow me up. I was so stupid and selfish. I had squandered Mum's precious energy on an insignificant niggle.

'How did it go?' Dad asked, turning on the engine.

'They couldn't do anything. Waste of time.'

I scanned the town as Dad drove home and replayed the earlier conversation with Mum in my head. *Real concern, not normal, needed sorting.* I should have understood what that really meant. If I'd known it would be like this, I wouldn't have bothered Mum, but I'd learnt my lesson. These pathetic struggles – nothing as important as Mum's ME – were to be shut away, repressed and ignored.

It must be normal then, I thought, to lie there for hour upon hour, wishing you could fall asleep pleasantly. Perhaps if I'd told Dr Hopkinson about the nightmares, it might have made a difference, but they felt too dark to mention. In those dreams I ran down the alleyway by my house, terrified that *It* would catch me. *It* was following me, running after me, close to taking me. I would fumble for the key and struggle to unlock my front door as *It* followed me up the driveway, seconds from grasping me. And then I'd wake up in a sweaty panic, alone in my bedroom. There was also the nightly recurring dream where a man held a gun to my head and asked me what I wanted to say before I died. But in those dreams, as in the surgery, I never had the right words.

Chapter Seven

Scarecrow

When I moved up to secondary school, I expected science lessons to be full of explosions, test tubes of green liquid transformed into blue, experiments that would blow my mind. But by Year 10 I'd learnt the main emphasis was on writing things down in a certain way. Our classroom was a dreary, windowless room with sets of four stools crowded around each desk containing a sink, which we never used. I peered over my work as our teacher, Mr Davis, wandered around the classroom whistling, his tie tucked into his shirt.

'Are you sure?'

'Definitely,' Jo whispered. 'He had an affair with a Year 11.'

'I can't believe it,' I said. Mr Davis was neither young nor attractive enough for me to think it possible.

'Both of them denied it,' Jo continued. 'But he left his wife for her and now they live together.'

She whipped her naturally blonde hair away from her face, inadvertently revealing an electric-blue bra strap. I didn't know where she bought her funky, push-up bras. Mine were limp, white bags from the old lady section in M&S, the only ones Mum allowed me to buy. I longed to go to town incognito and find flirty, rebellious underwear. I longed to fit in with my fifteen-year-old peers and not dress like a dowdy, middle-aged woman.

'When was this?' Rachel said.

'Only a few years ago.'

'How old's the girl now?'

'Maybe twenty. But that means he was at least in his thirties when she was in her teens.'

We pulled disgusted faces, unquestionably believing the school gossip, though it was impossible for me to know how much of it was the product of over-active teenage imaginations. We looked up in unison as Mr Davis leaned over a girl on another table, his arm around her shoulder.

'He's so creepy,' Carys said.

As Mr Davis stood up, we leant over our workbooks, fountain pens held in a meaningful position, though we'd finished our work long before.

My school was a vast jumble of interlinking buildings, each reflecting the era in which it was built. The science block was the most seventies of them all: a flat-roofed set of rooms connected with narrow hallways, the historic graffiti denting the walls.

'Did you read about the IRA ceasefire?' Carys said, her shoulder-length, black hair slicked back in a smooth pony-tail.

'It won't last,' Jo said. 'It never does.'

'I don't see how it'll ever end,' Rachel said, reapplying her lip balm. 'It's all such a mess.'

I watched them wordlessly as they spoke. I had no idea about any of this.

'I thought Clinton was visiting,' Carys said. 'Seems to think he can sort it out.'

'What a load of bollocks,' Jo said.

'Exactly,' Rachel agreed. 'Clinton thinks he can waft in, solve a complicated, centuries-old problem just by being American.'

I listened to them without any insight of my own to add. I felt as useless and stupid as ever. How did they get these opinions? How did they know this was happening?

'How are you lot getting on?' Mr Davis asked, sidling up beside Jo.

'Oh no,' she said under her breath, dropping her face beneath her hair. He stooped down, leaning his arm around her to rest on the table so she was entirely hemmed in, unable to escape his warm, smoky breath as he inspected her work.

'Very good,' he said, smiling in satisfaction as he walked away.

'Urgh,' Jo said, shivering. 'He's so gross.'

As the day was warm enough to eat lunch outside, we headed to the vast green of the sports field, spotted with pockets of teenagers who were using their blazers as makeshift picnic blankets. Rachel lay back in the sun, her dark tumble of ringlets cascading down her shirt. At the weekends she often wore huge, hooped earrings but today she had pretty studs. I wished I could pierce my ears, but it was another of those things Mum disallowed. I sat beside Rachel, squinting in the midday brightness, my legs tucked beneath me.

'You never said what happened with Gareth,' Jo said, taking a bite of a sandwich.

Rachel smirked, 'I told him I was busy.'

'You didn't!' I blurted. 'You turned him down?'

'Oh, he's fit,' Jo said. 'I'd snog him.'

Rachel crinkled her nose, 'No way.' She turned to Carys for back up.

'Don't ask me,' Carys said with a shrug. 'I fancy Jarvis Cocker.'

Their smooth, tanned legs were laid out in the sunshine, while I hid mine further beneath me. No wonder they had boys chasing them. I wished I was allowed to shave my legs. But Mum had said it would 'start an irreversible cycle'. I didn't know what that meant but it sounded terrible, and she knew best. Still, I hated this time of year when everyone could see my hairy legs. I wished I was more like my friends with their style and freedom and opinions. Instead, the girls in my form pushed me around, made fun of me and nicknamed me Scarecrow for my messy, ash-coloured hair, spotty skin and lack of make-up. I was an outcast, unable to fit in. Everyone else seemed to know how to grow up: how to style their hair, how to dress fashionably, how to revise, how to date, how to have intelligent conversation. I desperately tried to catch up with them, but I didn't know *how*. I felt like an ugly, pathetic mess and I hated myself for it. I chastised myself every evening for the stupid things I'd said at school and wished that I didn't exist.

'It's probably a good thing, Rach,' Jo said, her voice edgy with sarcasm. 'You don't want to end up pregnant, after all. Mr Travis would go mental.'

I don't know if it was Mr Travis's dark moustache, the shape of his face or his hairstyle, but he reminded me of Hitler. In his mid-forties with trousers up to his navel, he had taken on the unofficial role of school uniform monitor and was giddy with power. He purposefully stalked through the school, lurking as pupils walked through the corridors, ready to pounce on his next victim with their untucked shirt.

'I think our sex ed class will haunt me forever,' I said, shaking my head violently to dispel the memory.

'Fuck!' Carys blurted, and we spluttered on our lunch.

'That was the weirdest lesson ever,' Rachel laughed. 'If my dad knew Mr Travis had walked into the classroom shouting swear words, he'd go mental.'

'What was even the point?' I said, checking the field for teachers. 'To show us he knew the slang?'

'Maybe he hoped we'd think he was cool,' Carys said.

'Oh no,' said Jo, digging around in her bag. 'I forgot. Anyone got some tampons?'

'I've got some,' Rachel said.

They were a different species – these girls embracing womanhood – while I remained somehow trapped, a child in a woman's body. Mum had told me that she didn't use tampons and she had no intention of explaining to me how to use them. When I started my periods, she'd given me a maternity pad, presumably kept from my birth, twelve years earlier. These thick, mattress-size pads felt like a punishment for the misdemeanours forced upon me by my wayward body. Mum's comments were similarly targeted. She would burst into my bedroom as I was dressing and say, 'I see your pubic hair is coming along well,' and 'You've got larger breasts than me already.' Even three years later I felt embarrassed at the very thought of periods, puberty and growing up.

I squinted in the sunshine and saw Charlie walking across the grass with his blazer over his arm, his baby-blonde curtains brushing against his face as he approached. I sat up a bit taller, making sure my legs were out of sight. I wished I'd brushed my hair. He was panting as he reached us, his cherubim cheeks flushed red.

'You alright?' I asked.

'Not really. Just been caught by Travis.'

'Bad luck,' Rachel said, shaking her head.

'As if I don't have enough work to do, now I've got this stupid thing as well,' he complained plonking down beside me. He waved the small, blue sheet of paper with D-Merit printed in offensive, black capitals, demanding a two-page essay on the importance of a tidy uniform.

'You coming running later?' Carys asked.

'Yeah, alright,' said Rachel, brushing a curl behind her ear. 'I need to get my fitness up for D of E.'

'I don't think it counts when you stop every three minutes for a fag,' Charlie joked, a wicked grin curling his lips. Rachel gave him a sarcastic half-smile in return, and I watched his eyes work their way up from her long, bronzed legs.

The bell rang and we grabbed our things haphazardly, traipsing back across the field and through the labyrinth of buildings towards the maths block. I heard someone behind me shout my name – the authoritative voice of a teacher. It was sure to be Travis. I hurriedly tucked in my shirt, fumbling to hold my numerous bags and dropping my A2 art binder in the process. Gathering it up, I turned around to see Mr Reynolds, my unkempt English teacher, his dark beard bouncing as he marched towards me.

'Uh oh,' said Carys, walking on. 'Good luck.'

I waited for Mr Reynolds to catch me. 'Yes, Sir?'

'Fantastic sonnet,' he said stopping in front of me.

I took an unexpected breath in and spluttered a reply. 'Oh, thanks, Sir.'

'Well executed and the only one in the class to even attempt it. Good job. You've got an A.'

'Oh, thank you, Sir,' I said to his back as he strode away.

I stood there alone for a moment, certain I must be glowing as the sunshine beat warm on my back. It was a tiny spark of light that I knew I had to keep hidden, a treasure to store away in case anyone ruined it. My friends had turned the corner. I ran to catch them up.

When I got home that afternoon, Dad was brewing tea in the kitchen and Mum was upstairs in bed.

'Is it that time already?' she said, putting down her magazine as I went into her room.

She turned to get out of bed, extending one leg and then the other as if to admire their slender form. I sat down on the edge of her bed by the door while she scrutinised her face in her dressing-table mirror, adding some orange lipstick and pursing her lips. Standing and walking towards me, she paused by the scales. I knew what this meant. It was a regular and well-established routine, one that didn't need voiced instructions. I attentively took my place beside her. It was time to check our weight – or rather, my weight.

'Oh dear, eight stone one pound,' she said, leering down over me. 'I've never weighed more than eight stone in my whole life.'

I already knew this. She told me every time we stood here.

'I only weighed more when I was pregnant, and even then, I put on one stone and lost it as soon as I had you. Everyone said how tiny my bump was. I've shown you the photos before. But I didn't eat. Only nuts and dry biscuits the whole pregnancy.'

I kept my head bowed and wished I could rip the extra pound out of me. She was eight stone for her whole life and there I stood, fifteen years old, already weighing more than an adult woman. I hated myself, my disgusting fat body, my lack of self-control for eating too much.

Mum's slimness was one of her prized possessions, one of her boasts. She stood out amongst her family and her friends for being the tallest and the thinnest.

'It's so unfair,' Sandy had said to us once in her soft Geordie accent.

Sandy had been Mum's best friend since I was small, a glamorous lady who dressed in smart twinsets with perfect, soft strawberry blonde curls that floated around her face like candy floss.

'I want to be able to eat whatever I want and still be thin,' she said. 'It must be genetic.'

Mum beamed. 'It isn't. My parents were huge. But then they loved a daily fry-up. Not like me. I hate eating fat.'

'And look at you, pet,' Sandy said, turning to me with a teasing smile. 'Just like your Mam. It makes me want to spit.'

'She eats like a fly,' Mum said. She was pretending to be distressed by this statement but was unable keep her pleasure hidden. 'She doesn't even finish the smallest meals.'

I blushed, knowing that this was a double-edged compliment. Mum loved that I was underweight, but mealtimes were a battle-ground. I didn't like rice or pasta or potatoes. I didn't eat cake or biscuits either. I didn't enjoy eating at all. I felt alien, separated from my friends and their delight in cooking and eating and I worried about going on dates when I was older, like they did in *Friends*, because I couldn't finish a meal. It wasn't a choice not to eat; there was no fear of food or desire for control; I just didn't ever feel hungry. My mind had cut off the desire to eat, disassociated this sense, as if protecting me from the endless comments Mum made. I could easily skip a whole day's worth of meals without feeling a thing, but I was fragile for it. I couldn't run a loop of the school field without becoming faint, and every cold I caught floored me as if it were the flu. I didn't make the link between these weaknesses and my tiny calorie intake, instead scolding myself for not having the stamina of my peers.

'If we could take a pill, rather than eat food, then we would,' Mum had told Sandy. 'We can't help being thin. We can't help it if our favourite food is salad.'

The scales were showing over nine stone as Mum stepped off them, but I knew better than to comment. Mum was older and taller than me, so she was allowed to weigh more. But for me it was unacceptable. I chided myself for my greed. I despised myself.

Elinor's Diary

10th April 1998
Helen home from school. Tired depressed. Cried and we had chat about problems. Very difficult. Had martinis and bed.

13th May
Wet – up early took Helen to town. Got trousers in River Island. Home exhausted. Rang Sandy. Alan went out. Spent rest of day in bed except for meals. Helen very low in spite of trousers.

Chapter Eight

Failure

For two years I'd got home after school and hidden, crying until my face burned, chipping away at myself in the privacy of my bedroom. It was burying my fingernails into my skin until the impression didn't go and scratching my arms and knife cuts. It was plunging my face into ice-cold water in the bathroom sink and hoping I wouldn't take another breath. It was lying on the carpet of my bedroom, curled up in the foetal position, praying to God that I would die there and not have to feel like this any more. I was a failure as a daughter, I was a failure as a person: this was my mantra.

I don't know why I told Jo what I'd done. I don't remember the words I used to tell her, only that I said it with a half-smile, although neither she nor I found it funny. In the darkness of my bedroom it had seemed to make sense to try to end it. It was a poor attempt, and I was embarrassed, but I had meant it. I didn't want to exist any more.

And then, before I knew what was happening, Jo and I were in my head of house's office. Mrs Warburton was as warm and comforting as her name suggested, but sitting in the small room at the front of the hall, the door wide open as other pupils walked past on their way to lessons, I felt exposed and raw. Mrs Warburton was behind her desk facing us, her petite features framed with fly-away, straw-blonde hair.

'Jo tells me you tried to hang yourself last night, is that right?'

I nodded and tried to swallow down the half-smile that kept forming.

'That's not good, is it?' she said.

I stifled a sarcastic laugh. Jo had told us, in another science lesson, that she thought suicide was selfish, but she didn't understand either. It wasn't selfish if everyone would be better off without you.

'Why did you do it?' Mrs Warburton asked.

I shrugged. I didn't know what had created those feelings inside of me. I had a good life with good parents. I didn't want for anything. It was inexplicable that I hated myself to the point of destruction.

'Is it because you aren't a prefect?' Mrs Warburton said, laying her head to her shoulder.

I scoffed a little, 'No.'

'Because it doesn't mean you aren't a good pupil. Being a prefect is about having a certain skill set.'

'I know,' I said. 'I don't mind not being a prefect.'

'Are you being bullied?'

'I guess, a bit,' I said, thinking of the mocking comments, the name calling and the pushing around I received daily from the youths in my form.

We all fumbled on our seats. This explanation wasn't enough. I didn't have the words to explain that the bullies were only confirming what I already knew about myself – I was worthless – and Mrs Warburton didn't have the questions to dig any deeper. There weren't procedures to deal with a quiet middle-class girl who self-harmed, no certainty in what should be done.

'I'd like to inform your parents, if that's okay with you,' Mrs Warburton said. She read my panicked expression. 'But I don't have to tell them the details. Just that we had a chat today.'

A bag of marbles rolled in my stomach as I walked home that afternoon. My hands shivered as I unlocked the front door, and I crept in as if the floor were covered in needles.

'Good day?' Mum said. She was making herself tea in her post-nap, crinkled clothing.

'Not bad.'

'There's tea in the pot. Hurry, *Watercolour Challenge* is about to start.'

I poured the tea from the stainless-steel teapot and carried the cup through carefully, focusing on the saucer, the scalloped shape of the rim.

'Just in time,' she said, tapping the sofa seat.

I sat beside her and watched the contestants paint a landscape as we drank our tea, waiting for Mum to start the inevitable conversation. I waited, but nothing was said. No hint of displeasure or upset was given, not that day nor the next. I wondered if Mrs Warburton had called. Maybe she'd hoped that if she ignored the encounter, then the wordless teen would get over it.

I don't remember any conversations with Mum about my chat with Mrs Warburton, only that, several months later, I was going to see a counsellor. Dad always did the driving, but on this rare occasion it was just me and Mum, heading to a part of town I hadn't been to before. I don't remember what the counsellor looked like or what we talked about. I only remember what I didn't tell her:

I didn't tell her that I hated myself.
I didn't tell her that I self-harmed.
I didn't tell her that I couldn't sleep.
I didn't tell her that I felt like a worthless failure.
I didn't tell her that I wanted to die.
She didn't ask me about those things.

Afterwards, Mum picked me up alone. I clicked my seatbelt and we drove off, the streets melting away in the rear-view mirror and in my memory.

'You're all better now,' Mum declared.

I wrung my hands, picked at my nails and felt horribly ashamed of myself. I knew I had been selfish, pushing myself to the forefront when I should have been thinking about my poor mum. I wished I'd never said anything to Jo.

Elinor's Diary

17th July 1998
Helen to school. Alan and I to Safeway. Rest. Helen home quick change and I took her to counsellor. Came back in 1 hour. Helen seemed ok and doesn't want another appointment at the moment. Quiet evening.

24th July
Tried to rest without much luck. Helen to town, I to ME meeting. Was chairman, secretary and Treasurer and had 4 Visitors home 4:30. Helen home by 5 with stunning evening dress. We are in shock but she looks wonderful.

Chapter Nine

A Glimpse of the Fire

America was glorious. It was a new world where life was good. I'd seen it on American sitcoms and believed it was true, but at sixteen I saw it for myself.

During my final year at school, I'd tried to pull myself together, get over it, be better – just like Mum had told me to. I'd focused on doing things I enjoyed to forcibly be happy or, at the very least, make myself appear happy. I threw myself into activities, kept busy and fought the despair. And although I regularly wished I'd gone through with ending my life, I found that I could push those negative feelings down successfully.

I'd finished my GCSEs and the reward for all that work, all that positive thinking, was our 'once in a lifetime' family holiday to the States. My parents and I flew to Chicago, a monstrous city where everything was supersized. Our fifteenth-floor hotel room was so large that the two double beds swam in an ocean of space. I stood in the window and gaped at the city, so bright it appeared to be in flames. In Chicago we took the shotgun lift to the top of the Sears Tower and rode a Ferris wheel on Navy Pier, like a normal family having a fun time together.

Mum said that the heat in America made both my parents better and, though I saw Dad struggling for breath whenever we wandered out of the air conditioning, I believed her because life in the US was utterly different to normal. Dad was always around, only occasionally disappearing to the hotel bars in the afternoons. And Mum was completely better, no longer needing afternoon rests or struggling to walk. The only hint of disability was her insistence on having a wheelchair at the airport, but apart from that, we spent the entire two weeks racing from one activity to the next at a million miles an hour. There wasn't a pause, a rest or a complaint and Mum walked everywhere, block after block. We went to the theatre and to a ski run, to giant malls and water ski shows, museums and aquariums and planetariums. We ate at all sorts of stereotypical American eateries, from small diners straight out of a movie to Planet Hollywood. It was a lifetime of days out squeezed into a fortnight, and, best of all, for the first time in my memory my parents were well enough to enjoy it. It was my longed-for dream. America had cured them.

Chicago was only the starter. Most of the fortnight was spent in Wisconsin with my cousin, Cody, and his beautiful wife, Edith. Cody was a ball that had been bounced too hard, one that hurtled around with unbridled energy, nothing like the fifty-somethings I knew back in the UK. He looked like one of the Beach Boys with a white smile and bright blonde hair, his all-American wife with her perfect tan fawning by his side.

'This one's mine,' he grinned, rubbing his hand down the hull where the yacht bobbed on the edge of the lake. We'd driven there, the air conditioning up high, he and I chain-eating candy bars and singing along to 'What's the Story, Morning Glory', while my parents cringed in the back. Mum was in the only pair of shorts she owned, her ghost-white calves luminescent in the sunshine. She insisted on wearing a life-jacket on the boat, though none of the rest of us were, and she gripped onto the sides, her perm ruined by the wind as we flew over the water. Dad wore a huge smile as he recalled his own sailing days, his bum bag around his middle, his stomach bulging over the top.

'Hey, Helen, wanna go tubing?'

I hung onto the rubber ring for as long as I could, bouncing over the waves until my arms ached. When I finally let go and splashed into the water, I was horrified to see the boat fading into the distance. I floated in the water trying to talk myself out of panic while fish as large as Great Whites slid past my legs, the boat turning around far beyond me. When it returned, Cody heaved me back on board and I sat, wrapped in a towel, panting like a dog. We skirted the perimeter of the lake until he pulled up by a rock face, passing the controls to Edith and diving into the water.

'Where's he going?' I asked as he swam towards a cove.

Edith laughed, pointing to the top of the cliff a few seconds later as Cody waved at us, bombing thirty feet into the water and making the boat rock.

'Cody!' Edith yelled to him as he burst out of the waves, flicking his hair from his face. 'You're such a goof.'

I was in a TV show, an American sitcom, set amongst beautiful people and their perfect lives. My life in the UK had been a bad dream that I had seen in fuzzy monotone, but I had woken up to a technicoloured reality, one I didn't want to end.

'Anyone want ice cream?' Cody asked, climbing up the ladder at the back of the boat. 'We can swing by Dairy Queen on the way home.'

'Oh yeah,' Edith said. 'And when we get back, we could paint your nails, Helen.'

I loved the way she closed her eyes when she smiled, like she was the most contented person alive. She was pretty and enchanting, and she wanted to spend time with me. I adored her.

'Yeah,' I said, 'my nails are the longest I've ever had them right now. I haven't bitten them since we arrived. I'm so happy here.'

'Oh hardly,' Mum said, pulling down her sun hat. 'More like you don't have time to bite them.' The heartbeat of silence made sure I was deflated.

'I've got all sorts of colours,' Edith continued, bowing her head to pick up my dejected face. 'We could do anything.'

'Oh my goodness,' Mum said, pointing into the water. 'Look, a snake.'

It was tiny, shorter than my forearm, and was swimming along beside the boat. I could still feel the fish against my legs.

'Thank goodness I didn't go in,' Mum said with a fixed sneer.

I felt dozy back in the car, leaning on Mum, her skin cool from the air conditioning, not sticky with sweat and lake water like my own.

'Cody, could you drop me home on the way?' Edith said. 'I think I'm getting a migraine.'

Dairy Queen was my idea of heaven: a fast-food restaurant full of ice cream, frozen yogurt and sweets. Dad had a coffee that he drank with his face curled up, Mum refused to have anything.

'Whatcha gonna have?' Cody asked, elbowing me in the ribs playfully as we stood in the queue.

'I dunno,' I said, staring at the menu behind the counter. I couldn't make sense of the options. 'What are you having?'

'I'm thinking snickerdoodle cookie dough,' he said, and I laughed.

'I have no idea what that is,' I said, 'But I'll have the same.'

'Two snickerdoodles,' he said to the server. 'Both large.'

'No,' I said, grabbing his arm. 'I'll just have a small.' I didn't want to fail to eat it and waste Cody's money. I didn't want him to be disappointed in me.

'What?' Cody said, gawping at me with comic disgust. 'Don't be ridiculous.' He turned back to the server, 'Both large.'

'You're British!' the server said to me. He was seventeen at most, tall and athletic with dark eyes and a perfect smile. 'Are you from London?'

'No,' I said, smiling at Cody. 'I live in the countryside.'

'Your accent is so cute.'

Cody nudged my arm as we walked back to our table. 'Hey, he seemed into you,' he said. 'You should ask him out.' I could see Mum's narrowed eyes following me and hoped Cody would drop it before she was in earshot.

'What size are they?' Mum asked. I was melting quicker than the ice cream.

'It's got to be large,' Cody declared, putting an arm around me.

Mum leered as I took the first mouthful, pursing her lips tightly. I ate in clammed restraint as Dad and Cody talked, only daring to glance occasionally at the teenage server, imagining him bending down to kiss me, asking me to stay in America forever and be his girlfriend.

'Remember to be quiet. Edith's probably sleeping,' Cody said as we got back to his house, the late afternoon sun high in the sky. They lived in a bungalow that was identical to the one beside it, on a street that looked like every other on the block. The roads were wide and quiet, the yards flowing seamlessly into the next.

Dad and I slipped soundlessly into the house behind Cody, listening out for Edith and hearing nothing. The narrow hallway led into the kitchen-diner, the absence of a kettle jolting me each time we came in, as if to remind me that this wasn't my normal life. Cody headed down the corridor to the bedroom to see if Edith was well enough for dinner.

Mum was a fun fair behind us, slamming the front door as she came in. She was talking abnormally loudly, the vacuum of noise replaced by her full-volume chatter. Cody whipped round, his sunny demeanour replaced by a heavy glower. Dad glared at Mum, waving his arms frantically to hush her. She put her hand to her mouth, covering her Cheshire-cat smile in a faux apologetic stance. Dad and Cody walked away, but I was petrified to the spot, unable to turn away. I'd witnessed something catastrophic, something unbelievable, and I couldn't move on.

It's not that big a deal, I told myself. *She forgot to be quiet, that's all. It's not a big deal.*

I wanted to believe it, to walk away and forget it. But it was a big deal. It was a huge slap in the face. I'd spent every afternoon of my childhood making myself invisible so I didn't disturb Mum. I'd had years of long weekends when my self-sufficient entertainment had to be muted so that I didn't inconvenience her. I'd compromised everything about myself so she could rest. But Mum couldn't keep quiet for two minutes to do the same for someone else. Edith had welcomed us into her home and cared for us. She'd taught me to play the piano and spent time with me – something that had never happened before. But Edith wasn't important enough for Mum to keep quiet. My cheeks were burning, but I couldn't tell if it was with embarrassment or anger or betrayal.

Mum pushed past me to go into Cody's lounge, and I stood in the kettle-less kitchen trying to regain my balance. It was a crack in *The Matrix* that I couldn't quite make sense of – a moment when my idol's clay feet were revealed. But that didn't mean she was no longer my idol. I shook my head, pushed the thoughts down and followed her. Whatever had happened I couldn't speak it. I had to keep it in.

Chapter Ten

Breaking Chains

I rushed between the oven, chopping board and fridge, the heat of the kitchen adding to my frazzled appearance. If I'd had any cooking experience, I'd have known this was a mistake, but I was far too stubborn to give in. The kitchen was new: an extension forced through by my parents despite my protestations. Apparently it didn't matter that it was my last year at home before university. It didn't matter that studying for my A levels would be backdropped by builders' radios blaring and the noise of construction work. It wasn't necessary for us to have a kitchen for my final Christmas before I left home. And, according to my parents, my suggestion that they hold off their dream home for a year was selfish.

'This isn't your house!' Dad had shouted at me, and it certainly wasn't after that.

The extension had doubled the size of the kitchen, but it was as messy as it ever had been, every counter space crammed with utensils and cooking equipment. Mum still didn't cook.

'I don't know how you're going to cope at university.'

She'd said it so often in the last year, it had become wearing, the sharp spike of mockery digging a little deeper every time.

'You can't cook, you can't do your own washing. I don't know what you're going to do.'

It was repeated to me, to her friends, to relatives on the phone. I was fed up with hearing how useless I was.

'You've never shown me how to cook,' I countered, feeling every inch the obnoxious teen, facing her with my hands on my hips, my highlighted hair held back from my face in miniature plaits. I wanted to be able to speak to her sensibly, but she goaded me. I hated that my sulky responses seemed to prove her point.

'You won't let me teach you,' she said, throwing her hands into the air.

Since she'd never offered to show me how to cook, I'd never had the opportunity to turn her down. It was the same with cleaning and washing and shopping and managing money – I wasn't expected or asked to do any chores, and I didn't think to offer to do them. It was a luxurious existence that lulled me into a confused sense of identity. Was I lazy? Was I spoilt? I couldn't complain about my life because I was so privileged, yet I felt a leaden responsibility on my shoulders: an inexplicable burden of care for my parents that had no obvious actions attached. The daily tidying away of my needs and feelings and desires to prioritise my parents was a duty so ingrained that it would take another two decades for me to identify it.

'As I told Sandy,' Mum continued, 'You're going to starve.'

'I can cook,' I said, my temper rising. 'It's not difficult to follow a recipe.'

'Oh really?' she said, in that sarcastic voice, the one that told me I was a silly, petulant child who didn't know what I was talking about.

'Why don't I cook for you and Dad tomorrow?'

She crossed her arms over her coffee-coloured blouse, letting her head drop to one side as if I were suggesting the impossible.

'Go on then.'

'Alright, I will. A three-course meal.'

'Oh, right!'

The last time I'd made anything that didn't go in the microwave it was a cake I baked with Mum when I was four. Apart from helping Carys cook once, when I mistakenly thought you mashed the potatoes before you cooked them, I had no kitchen experience. Literally not a sausage. That night I read through the recipe books on the shelves and designed the meal, choosing foods we'd never eaten at home before, not realising that I was making the task unnecessarily difficult. I was determined to impress them. I wanted to make it clear I didn't need them.

I was still wearing an apron as I brought the bruschetta into the dingy dining room the following evening, taking a seat between my parents on the mahogany and black vinyl chairs.

'Enjoy,' I said, the plates illuminated by a dim yellow light.

The cutlery clattered and scraped, the noise bouncing around the walls. I took a bite keeping my expression level and my head bowed though the tomatoes were exploding like fireworks in my mouth. I knew better than to give any indication that the meal was a success. I trembled as I cleared up the empty plates, making sure I didn't catch Mum's sour stare, returning with lasagne, then apple pie, the clatter of the plates and silverware the only sound. Watching out of the corner of my eyes, continuing to keep my head down, I saw Mum chewing with exaggerated motion. She was blinking rapidly, and I knew that, despite the soggy bottom on the pie, I'd proved her totally, utterly wrong. She sucked in her cheeks as I cleared the bowls away, pushing back her chair intently.

'Now you've done it once, you can do it more often,' she announced, striding away from the table.

Hidden in the kitchen, loading the dishwasher, I allowed myself to smile. Mum had expected burnt toast and beans, not homemade pastry. She'd envisaged laughing with her friends at my teenage bravado. She was waiting for me to fail and crawl back to her, apologetically admitting I needed her help. She didn't seem to realise that I'd learnt to rely on myself a long time before.

Chapter Eleven

Escape

'What's wrong?' Mum said.

I was sitting on the unused chair in the lounge, biting my nails and blankly staring out of the window as the late summer sun dropped down towards the horizon. It hadn't been properly hot that year, only warm enough to trick me into shorts and vest tops that left me goose pimpled.

'Bit worried about tomorrow.'

'Why?'

She stood over me in her camel-coloured shirt dress, buttoned to the waist with a pleated skirt. It was so unfashionable, so out of touch.

'It's my A-level results,' I said, pulling a contemptuous teenage sneer.

She flashed her eyes at the ceiling. 'I know that.'

I examined one of my nails, short and lopsided, the skin peeling at the side. If she knew, then why was she asking me?

'Don't be worried.'

I dragged my eyes to glance up at her. 'It's not that simple though, is it? If I don't get two As, I won't get into Nottingham. Or any of my uni choices. So then it'll be clearing, which'll be stressful.'

'It'll be fine,' Mum said, walking towards the door. 'You don't need to be worried. I never expected you to go to university anyway.'

I sat up and turned in the seat to face her. 'What do you mean? That's always been the expectation.'

'No, it hasn't,' she said, spinning round in her flat, cream drivers. 'Me and your dad didn't go, so I wouldn't expect it from you.'

I rubbed my face. 'But you said my primary teacher told you that I was bright enough to go to uni and you and Dad have been saving for me to go ever since.'

She shrugged as if it was another thing I'd made up. 'I suppose you're right.'

Maybe she'd read somewhere that you shouldn't put too much pressure on your children and thought she was practising good parenting. But it felt like she was purposefully contradicting me, dismissing my feelings again, forcing me to swallow emotions she didn't want me to express.

Mum and Dad hadn't seemed that interested in me going to university. They'd given little support as I'd studied for my A levels and, while many of my school friends engaged in typical teenage experimentation, I only dipped my toe in, determinedly focused on getting good grades and taking extra tuition to ensure it. Mum's input in my application to universities had been to furiously accuse me of being a difficult teenager, criticise my ability to live alone and veto my top choices – both London and York were apparently too far away from home. Dad had taken me to a few open days, but I'd been left to research and fill in my UCAS form alone. My parents were emotionless bystanders to what felt like the biggest event of my life.

I couldn't face breakfast the morning of my results. I checked the clock every five minutes for five hours and thanked God that my dad insisted on leaving early. I was jittery, my palms sweaty. I gripped the piece of paper, trying not to smudge the university phone numbers I'd carefully copied down. They were in order of desirability with clearing at the bottom, ready for my inevitable failure.

Mum, Dad and I walked from the car park into the throng of anxious students and their families, Dad choosing to stand near the ramped entrance, leaning on the handrail and pulling his inhaler from his buff utility waistcoat. My stomach churned. My friends and acquaintances fidgeted around me, some with edgy, serious faces, others in a state of hyperactivity. I couldn't believe I was there. Dad hadn't dropped down dead. I hadn't become Mum's full-time carer. I stood on the precipice of a new life out of the shadow of my parents' needs and disabilities.

The doors opened and I went into the large, cool hall with my peers, all of us trying not to appear too keen. We queued behind tables heavy with boxes of alphabetically ordered envelopes, the teachers behind the desks flicking through the names. I was giddy and giggly, dancing around beside Charlie as he fidgeted, repeatedly pulling his hands through his newly cut, blonde hair.

'What do you need?' I asked.

'AAB. You?'

'Same. Why is it so slow? Just grab the envelope and go guys.'

'They need to hurry along before I wet myself,' he said, joining in my Riverdance as we edged towards the front of the queue.

As it was given to me, the plain, brown envelope burned in my hands, full of promise and trepidation. Charlie and I stood at the edge of the hall and stared at each other as we pulled out the single sheet of paper with our results.

'I can't read it,' I said, my eyes skipping from letter to letter, incapable of making any sense of the words. I couldn't focus, couldn't understand it.

'I did it,' Charlie said. 'AAB!'

'No way!' I gasped, grabbing his arm too tightly. 'Me too!'

There was a blinding flash, a moment of relief and disbelief, a climatic explosion of emotions. I threw my arms around Charlie, almost crying but laughing too, so wrapped up in myself that I was unable to register he was hugging me back.

'I can't believe we did it!'

That thin, white paper was the invitation to a life of my own, a future away from my parents and my little home town. I pulled back from Charlie and examined the letter again, fearing I'd misread. I'd really done it. The room was heady with excitement and disappointment, a fragile cocktail that would be followed up with alcoholic comfort later. I couldn't believe it. I stumbled through my friends towards my parents, walking on a soft cloud of success.

'Look,' I said, passing them the results. 'Look!'

'What, what… I don't understand it,' Mum stuttered, snatching the paper from my hands.

'I got it! Two As and a B.'

'And an A in General Studies,' Dad said, tapping my back and smiling.

'Oh my god,' Mum breathed.

She grasped the handrail and bent her knees to make it seem like she was fainting.

'Oh my god.'

'Pull yourself together, Elinor,' Dad hissed, his cheeks turning red, shifting frantically in the hope that no one else could see her display.

'I can't believe it,' Mum said, wiping a limp hand across her forehead. Dad was grabbing her arm and pulling her up forcefully. I couldn't see straight.

'Is it that much of a surprise?' I said, wrinkling my nose. It was a crashing comedown from the riot of delight in the hall. 'I thought you said I shouldn't worry. It would be fine.'

'But I didn't expect it,' Mum said, leaning heavily onto Dad. 'I didn't expect AAB.'

I felt breathless, like I needed to sit down, too many emotions rushing around my head.

'I needed AAB to get into Nottingham,' I said.

'Yes, yes,' she said, shooing me away with a flick of her hand.

I laughed at her reaction, believing she was as overwhelmed and thrilled as I was, even if it left me feeling awkward and uneasy, the brightness of my success tarnished.

Elinor's Diary

16th August 2001
Helen up 5:30. Had breakfast 7:30. Helen so nervous. 10:30
we all went to college. In by 10:50 and Helen got AAB
Amazing – she was in shock. We went home and opened
champagne.

Chapter Twelve

Honey Pot

It was eternal autumn at university – a mix of cool days and raincoats, the summer, Easter and Christmas stolen by the long holidays. Despite Mum's reservations I enjoyed living alone. For once in my life, there was only me, my needs and my feelings to worry about.

'Six weeks you've been gone,' Mum said to me, her voice fiery with outrage, when I returned home. 'Six weeks!'

'That is what I told you I'd do,' I said. 'I needed to settle in.'

'But six weeks!'

At home we had a cleaner and a gardener, my dad did all the cooking and, unlike my friends, as a teenager I wasn't asked to do chores. I'd never done a load of washing, gone to the supermarket alone, put out the bins or cleaned a toilet, and I didn't have the skills to care for myself. I see now it was a devious form of neglect: my parents failed to give me the knowledge I needed and then mocked me for not having it. From the outside, it looked like I was spoiled, but my parents weren't preparing me for life away from them, perhaps because I wasn't supposed to go.

At uni I was teaching myself how to cook and clean and live independently, whilst also negotiating a new city, new living arrangements and a university degree amongst complete strangers. I was overwhelmed. My parents had done little to help me prepare for university, and I felt desperately out of my depth. I remember sitting on my bed a week into my first term, weeping into a catalogue of seminars, with no idea what I was doing.

Despite disorganised flapping around for several weeks (or, debatably, three entire years) I not only managed to feed myself and keep vaguely clean, but also succeeded at my degree. History students only had four hours of lectures a week and we were expected to be self-disciplined enough to spend most of our time in the library studying under our own steam. I found all those afternoons I'd spent alone during my childhood meant I was already trained to be self-motivated in isolation. I had successfully escaped to my own life.

While I was in Nottingham, Carys was having her own uni adventure in Wales. We'd drifted apart during sixth form and, though I still enjoyed her company, we now only saw each other during the long holidays when we returned home.

Our leaving for university had coincided with Mum's relapse of ME. Though I believed her when she told me this, I couldn't see any marked difference from Mum's previous version of ME except that she didn't visit me in Nottingham. She only saw my hall of residence once and didn't see my student house – where I spent my second two years – until my final term. Though his health was worsening, Dad alone drove me back and forth from uni. He was the one who came to get me when I had chickenpox. He was the one I called in an emergency.

Still, things were easier once I was living apart from Mum. I'd spent most of the last year at home feeling like she was constantly provoking me to arguments to prove what a terrible teenager I was. But once I moved away, she was at the end of the phone whenever I needed her, and I felt the special relationship that we'd shared in my early teens had returned.

It was sunset, a clandestine hour when fierce apricot streaks were fading into peachy darkness. As I walked over the footbridge towards the engineering library, the cars below shot yellow beams into the half-light, illuminating the stream of students walking towards me on their way home. No one knew where I was or what I was doing because nothing was yet official.

I'd met Peter through friends, our flirtations over the pool table turning to late-night conversations as he walked me home from the pub, sharing concerns about our father's mutual heart problems. I'd quickly fallen for his sharp features and buzz cut, how easily he understood what it was like to have a dad whose health teetered on the edge, his quiet sensitivity. All Mum knew was that we were friends, but I must have mentioned his name a few too many times.

'I knew they'd be buzzing round you, like bees around a honey pot,' she'd said. It felt like she was talking about someone else. I couldn't imagine anyone wanting me: fat and stupid, ugly and unlovable. I'd gone home the weekend before, regretting it as soon as I walked through the door.

'Do you miss your lover?' she'd said to me, her devilish grin mocking her pathetic, love-struck nineteen-year-old. 'Do you love him?'

I'd walked away hoping she'd drop it, but the taunts had followed me all weekend. And then, the last evening before I'd returned to uni, she'd cornered me on the landing as I headed to bed. I was already in my pyjamas, she in a shiny polyester nightie edged in lace that skimmed the floor. She was close, forcing me to back up against my bedroom door.

'You haven't had sex with him, have you?'

Her hair was up in curlers, her face greasy with thick moisturiser and smelling of Oil of Ulay.

'No,' I said. 'We're just friends.'

'Well, you mustn't,' she insisted, her piercing eyes on me. 'Goodness knows what would happen to you. You could get AIDS and die. Or even worse, you could get pregnant.'

Her nostrils flared as she leant in towards me, pinning me to the spot, her breath on my face.

'It would ruin your life,' she said.

Her menacing glare was cemented onto me as she stepped away, remaining until she disappeared into her bedroom. I scurried into my own room, holding the handle to prevent her from following me. Was that conversation about her fear of me losing my virginity? Or was she telling me I'd ruined her life? I waited until I heard her own door close and then got into bed. It was much easier when we spoke on the phone.

I'd made sure she didn't know I was going out with Peter that night. The spring evening was warm so I wore a pink hoodie and a light denim skirt that flared above my knee. I ran down the steps on the other side of the bridge, weaving through the deserted engineering buildings, shadows creeping across the path. The further into the university I went, the quieter it was, like a deserted town where once there was life. I saw Peter from a distance sitting on a low wall in light-brown chinos and a navy-blue shirt, rolled up at the elbows.

'Hey,' he said, standing up as I got near. 'Fancy a walk?'

We headed up to the café and bought a couple of cans of lemon Coke, then skipped down the hill to the lake. The lights illuminated the water's edge, the pathway dipping into darkness.

'I'm not sure I fancy walking through the trees,' I said. 'Can we sit here instead?'

The bench overlooked the tranquil lake, the boats tied to one side, the ducks and swans floating inaudibly.

'It's so nice here,' I said, and he turned to me with his ice-blue eyes.

'Isn't it?' he agreed, and kissed me for the first time, his soft lips on mine.

When we walked back up the hill, we could see the whole university and the city beyond, glimmering in the night. This was only a snatched moment between lectures and revision for the upcoming exams. We walked home, through the quiet streets lit up by rows of desk lamps glowing in the windows of student houses, and he left me at my door. It had only been a few weeks, but I already knew that this was the man I was going to marry.

Chapter Thirteen

Broken

It happened on the morning of my final exam and continued, on and off, for the next four years. I was revising, and something clicked in my head like a switch being turned off. It was so palpable that I stopped and tried to shake it out of my head. But the huge grey cloud had already encompassed me, fogging my sight and remaining there when I dressed, as I put on my engagement ring, when I revised, when I took my exam, when I met Peter afterwards. It was there all day, a disconnect to the world, as if I was standing to the side of myself. That day I should have felt nervous and then relieved to have finished my degree – but what I actually felt was nothing. I knew the agony of self-loathing – the inescapable pain that had eaten me from within when I was in my teens – but this was different. This was a long, empty numbness.

The Christmas before, I'd found Dad collapsed in my parents' kitchen. He'd been unable to breathe, his already restrained lungs worsened by a bout of pneumonia, and had blacked out, smashing his head in the fall. A few months later he'd had a risky but necessary operation. All my fears were coming true at the wrong moment. Becoming Mum's carer didn't fit into taking exams and applying for jobs and getting married and having my own life.

Dad had stabilised and, now my exams were finished, the long summer lay in front of me, ready to be embraced before real life began. But the fear didn't leave me; it sank into thick blackness instead. And, though I wanted to feel brighter, I woke every day feeling empty, unable to shake it. I tried to cheer myself up by doing the things I loved, but this time it didn't make any difference. I was changed. I wrote it out – a description of the new me:

No feelings.
Nothing makes me happy.
No appetite.
Easily irritated.
Really, really tired.
Can't concentrate.

The doctor's surgery on campus was in the basement, the sun falling from the skylights in the waiting room and haloing the students' heads. I took deep breaths to try to slow my breathing, hiding my shaking hands in my pockets and only removing them to wipe the sweat onto my jeans. I knew this was not a safe place. Here there would only be suspicion and derision. There was no good outcome; either I would be dismissed as a time-waster or diagnosed as broken. But there was nowhere else to go. The tinny electronic voice called my name as the room number flashed on a computer screen and I stumbled to the end of the corridor. I was crying before I entered, passing the doctor the list, unable to speak. The doctor seemed unmoved. It was another classic case.

Depression wasn't something I'd even considered. I'd heard the word, my understanding limited to Eeyore or having a bad day and, while I'd have quickly snapped up medication for something physical, I was easily persuaded to wait before starting anti-depressants, as if this illness might clear up of its own accord given time. I left the surgery clutching a handful of leaflets with no more understanding of what was happening to me and no help on the horizon. I went back to my student house, packed up my belongings and returned home for the three-month summer holiday.

The cloud didn't lift when I went home. I was engulfed by relentlessly dull skies, though my parents didn't comment even when

I told them what the doctor had said. I wandered like a zombie, unable to find peace or make plans, though my wedding was just a few months away.

'I've always felt like this.'

I hadn't meant to say anything, but as we passed on the landing – Mum heading for her afternoon rest – it leapt out of me, refusing to be ignored.

'Like what?' she sighed, slumping in the doorway. She held her tea close to her chest, tapping her fingers on the china.

'Like, I dunno. Like I really dislike myself. I feel a bit... of a failure.'

'Oh,' Mum said, dusting her shoulder. 'That's strange.'

I examined the wallpaper carefully, each textured cream swirl, hoping Mum would say something to fill the emptiness. She didn't.

'It's been the same since I was... young,' I added, hoping to prompt her.

'I remember you being quite sad at school,' she said.

Quite sad. Did that mean she remembered speaking to Mrs Warburton? Did she see the knife cuts? Did she overhear my nightly tears? If she had, she hadn't done anything about it.

'You're not going to hurt yourself, are you?'

'No,' I said, quickly. 'I did when I was at school. But I won't now.' I scanned my socked feet, following the paisley pattern of the carpet with my toes. 'Have you ever felt like this?'

'No,' she said, the word ringing in my ears. 'No, I don't know where that's come from.' She pulled herself up as if to leave, fanning out her skirt. 'It certainly isn't anything to do with me. Sounds like there's something wrong with you, something inside.'

She started to walk into her room and then stopped, leaving me staring at her hunched back. 'Don't tell Dad though, will you? It would break his heart.'

The landing wasn't large, but it felt like it: a huge empty void, like the one inside me.

Chapter Fourteen

Fat

When I was thirteen, there was a night I couldn't sleep. I slunk downstairs in the darkness, carefully missing the squeaky steps and squeezing through gaps in the doors. It made me jump to see Dad awake, sitting in his chair in the lounge, unable to sleep either. I remember he wrapped me in a blanket, and we tiptoed into the garden. The sky of the countryside was a perfect deep black, and he showed me the stars, pointing out constellations and planets. It lasted no more than ten minutes, but it was one of my best moments with Dad.

The night before my wedding, I gazed up at the same sky alone, knowing that the next day everything was going to be different. The surprise was that it wasn't only the big stuff that changed – my name, where I lived, who I lived with – but all the little details. I could finally sleep. There were no more nightmares, no men with guns chasing me, no last words. I felt safe beside Peter. And I was eating and enjoying it, finishing meals without feeling I'd undergone a trial. Food didn't taste bland, inedible or stressful any more. Cake wasn't dry, chocolate biscuits were delicious, sausages and steak and burgers weren't mountains to be conquered but treats to be savoured.

'You were so thin,' Mum purred, as we reviewed my wedding photos. I'd felt like a princess in my sleeveless white gown, a cascade of sparkles running from my waist to the floor. 'I've seen other slim brides and they look sickly. But you looked gorgeous. You made everyone spit. They were sick with jealousy.' She turned her head to me, eyebrows arched. 'How much do you weigh now?'

'I'm nine stone,' I said, my voice low. The weight piled on and I didn't know how to stop it. I was out of control.

'Oh my goodness,' she gasped, examining me with an open mouth. 'Is that a size sixteen?'

I wrung my hands. 'No, I'm a size ten.'

'You can't be,' she said, smoothing her stomach. 'I'm a size ten.'

She turned the page on the wedding album and smiled at a close-up of her hands tying my corseted wedding dress.

'I showed Doris down the road the photo I took last time you came, and she said you look much better now,' she said, pausing for effect. 'She said you were far too thin at your wedding.'

To anyone else's ears, this would have sounded like a compliment. To really understand her meaning though, you'd have to know that Mum hated Doris. She thought she was an idiot, and her opinion wasn't just worthless, it was wrong. The translation was, 'Doris, who is a moron, thinks you look better now you're fat.'

I no longer saw the expressions of the people in the photographs or admired their clothes. Instead, I was assessing their waistlines to see if they were thinner than me. I couldn't see them, or myself, properly any more. All I could see was how horribly obese I had grown, my skin like melting wax as it folded over my stomach. I was so ashamed of myself.

Chapter Fifteen

Exhaustion

I didn't fit into the workplace, or that's what I told myself. After university, I worked as an admin assistant and then got a civilian job in the police, a well-paid and prestigious role I was only too proud to tell my friends and family about. The title didn't quite match the work though; I found it repetitive, dull administration, searching through databases and filling in forms. I was one of only five women who worked in the large office and felt out of my depth in the banter. When one of my male colleagues – a short, hook-nosed man in his fifties who insisted we call him 'Vic' though that wasn't his name – announced to the office that he'd been to the University of Life, I'd sink in my seat, only too aware that I'd swanned into a role with a good salary at twenty-two because I'd got a degree.

I didn't understand this world, the close-knit family of the police where civvies were merely tolerated. I didn't appreciate that still, in the early 2000s, there were only a scattering of female officers who had fought and sacrificed to get to their positions, while the majority of women in the force were working in secondary, civilian roles. I didn't know how to deal with the heavy weight of masculine bravado that hung in the air. It was only when I saw Vic lying across a desk in front of a young, blonde girl – no more than twenty years old – from HR, one knee bent up so his crotch was in her face, that I realised he regularly intimidated women. It was only then I understood that when he read the paper over my shoulder – leaning over me, his breath on the back of my neck – it was *meant* to unnerve me. That's why he waited until we were alone in the office. That's why, when

I offered him the paper to make him go away, he'd say he didn't want it. I didn't know how to deal with him beyond scooping the congealed brown sugar into his tea every time I brewed. It gave me a certain satisfaction even if I couldn't take the matter further. He wasn't the only male police officer in the office to act like this and I knew I wouldn't be taken seriously if I complained.

Dad was getting worse. He had chronic kidney disease and unruly diabetes and had lost huge amounts of weight inexplicably. His lungs were working at such a low capacity that he was wired up on oxygen 24/7 and could only have a few minutes away before he was unable to breathe. His dilated cardiomyopathy, a serious heart disease, had caused a run of heart attacks that meant ambulance dashes to hospital to be resuscitated. Peter and I had spent two years being woken by 4 a.m. phone calls telling us to come now, and we'd drive the hundred miles in the semi-darkness praying that Dad would hang on for one more hour. Each time, we arrived wondering if he'd still be alive, only to be told the storm had passed. But that was what heart disease was like, a nurse had told me: a rollercoaster ride where one moment the patient was critical and the next they were stable.

My friends were working towards their next promotion or were starting to try for a baby, but I was clinging on for dear life. It was only a matter of time until Dad died and then what? It was an unthinkable fear, impossible to verbalise. I remember sobbing to Peter that Dad's death would mean I would lose everything, without any understanding of what I meant. I was grappling with this visceral reaction that made no sense to me. After all, I might be losing my dad young, but I wasn't a child and I wouldn't lose *everything*. I couldn't grasp that my greatest fear was to return to the prison I'd only recently escaped. I thought Dad's death would mean I'd become Mum's carer, swallowed again into the world of her needs.

I was exhausted.

The tiredness consumed me. After all those years of struggling with insomnia, I was now faced with the opposite. It was as if my brain was shutting down, my eyes refusing to remain open, sucked into a vortex I couldn't escape. It was impossible to work full time, so I dropped my hours. I'd drive home at lunch time, quickly and unconsciously eat and then fall, zombie-like, into bed, waking two or three hours later. I'd make dinner ready for Peter's return from work and spend a quiet evening with him before gratefully falling back into bed in the evening. I felt weak, pathetic, unable to think straight or make decisions. And I was seeing things – spiders the size of dinner plates climbing up the walls, people who disappeared when I looked closely. I heard a crowd of laughing voices in a vacant office, a baby crying in my empty house, a meow next to me so loud it woke me up though we didn't have a cat. I knew these things weren't real and yet there they were, solid and tangible. And though the doctor merely put it down to needing my eyes testing, I thought I was going insane.

I saw multiple counsellors, but nothing I said in the sessions shed any light on why I felt like I did – wracked with catastrophized fears; filled with self-loathing; terrified to confront those who overstepped boundaries; doubting my every move, my every word, my every breath. The consecutive therapists I saw only seemed to watch in open-mouthed confusion, no more able to understand or explain what was happening inside of me to cause these debilitating emotions than I was. Their lack of help only proved Mum was right – I was broken, I was bad, I was failing.

It wasn't the most auspicious start and I thought Peter must have regretted marrying me, though he says he never felt that way. We are opposites: he's an engineer and I'm a creative. He's practical and logical and likes nothing more than a DIY project. I'd happily read the paper and write all day. Our house is full of Peter's sports equipment and my guitars. I make the mess, and he cleans up behind me. I'm chronically early, and he's always late. We often joke that had we lived together first, we'd never have got married.

Our overlap comes in our aspirations. We like eating out, going on holiday and cycling together but most of all we wanted a family and we wanted to cherish it. We both dreamt of the children we would have and the life we would give them, full of fun and love and happiness. But in the middle of our twenties, we were nowhere near starting our own family. Not only was Dad seriously ill, but I was quietly falling apart.

The GP I saw had an Irish accent, his patchy beard matching his flyaway blonde hair. I said I had depression. He asked for my symptoms. As I listed them, I could see him looking through me, barely listening. But was that real, or was that the paranoia? He turned to Peter who had come on my insistence. Was I crying already?

'What do you think is her main symptom?'

Peter shuffled in his seat. He'd come to support me, not to talk to the doctor on my behalf.

'I suppose, from my point of view, she sleeps a lot.'

'Sleeps a lot? Yes, you see,' he said turning back to me, 'this isn't depression. This is ME.'

I spluttered out a laugh. 'No. No this isn't ME. This is depression. I've had it before. I know. My mum has ME. I know what ME looks like.'

'Ah, there you are, see! Your Mum has ME. It runs in the family.'

No, I didn't have ME. I couldn't have ME. I knew he was wrong, but it still filled me with horror. He was incorrect – my symptoms pointed to depression with a dose of psychosis – but I was spending inordinate amounts of time in bed and the parallels with Mum were deeply unnerving. Every afternoon I went for a rest, just like she did, just like she had for two decades. It was too close for comfort. I didn't want to be like Mum. I didn't want to spend my time in bed. I tried to stay up, I tried to push through, but I was devoured by the emotional exhaustion, unable to fight it.

'It might seem like a silly question,' said one of my female colleagues, 'but have you thought about suicide?' She had long, perfectly straight hair and ate homemade salads for lunch. She was thin and attractive and successful and didn't understand. When I nodded, she tutted.

'I just don't know why. I know people in much worse situations than you and they're not considering suicide.'

I started looking for a part-time job. It was only admin, no big title this time, organising college students three days a week in an office full of women under thirty. My colleagues were calm and kind and the office had a totally different atmosphere. I spent my free time going to the gym and I began to get better. I stopped hearing things, I stopped seeing things, I didn't need to sleep all the time. But Dad's health was worsening still; there was little more the doctors could do and his prognosis was grim. Even my part-time job was too much for me and I left after a year. If I was ever going to be myself again, I needed time and space to recover.

Chapter Sixteen

Jigsaw Pieces

Mum was getting ready, the Sunday morning light pouring through the window as she sat at her dressing table. Peter and I had travelled to my parents' for the weekend, fearing that it might be *the* weekend. I'd tried to see as much of Dad as I could in those last two months, while he was in hospital permanently. His grip on reality was loosening every time I saw him as his breathing deteriorated and the oxygen reaching his brain ebbed. His heart was failing, and it was only a matter of time.

'I'm so tired,' I said, my shoulders slumped. I'd thrown on some grey cords that bulged around my stomach, bloated with a hunger that grew the more depressed I became. 'I'm exhausted.'

'I know,' Mum said, catching me in the mirror as she reapplied her make-up. 'Me too.'

'I don't know how much more of this I can do.'

My words stung on my lips. It was a betrayal of Dad to speak them. After all, this wasn't about me. He was the one suffering, the one facing death. It could be weeks, or it could be months and that thought made me feel desperate.

'I don't know how much more I can do either,' Mum said, coming to sit beside me and hanging a loose arm around my waist.

'I want this to be over, but if it's over…' I said, my voice trailing away.

'I know. One day at a time, that's all we can do.'

We drove to the hospital with Peter, getting there early so we could have a coffee before we visited. Once we had seen Dad, Peter and I would be heading back to Nottingham, ready to start the whole routine again. The cafe was empty, the metal chair cold on my back, the dodgy brown liquid scorching. There was nothing left to say, so I blankly scanned the hospital reception that had become far too familiar. Mum's mobile started to buzz from deep within her bag.

'Hello? Hello?' she said, fumbling the phone to her ear. She stood up before she hung up, stumbling out of her seat. 'It's the ward, we've got to go.'

'What?' I blurted, kicking back my own chair and grabbing her arm. 'What did they say?'

'He's taken a turn for the worse.'

I didn't know, at twenty-five, that this was medical code. I didn't know that death isn't dealt with honestly, even in hospitals, but is cloaked in gentle phrases that don't even touch on the reality. I'm not sure how this helps anyone. We raced up the stairs, even Mum not pausing at the lift. I ran ahead, taking the steps three at a time then skidded to a halt at the entrance to the ward, afraid of what I would find inside. Mum pushed past me, the nurse waiting for us by the door to Dad's side room.

'I'm so sorry,' she said.

I had been ready for this moment for fifteen years, since I'd overheard that Dad could drop dead at any time, but none of my imagined scenarios matched this. It happened in slow motion, my numb tears clouding my vision. Mum was falling: a carefully controlled crumple that meant the nurse and I grabbed her before she could kneel on the floor. She was wailing loudly, her mouth open wide though her face was dry. We pulled her onto a nearby chair and she continued howling while I stood by, a bewildered and uncomfortable observer. I imagined being a patient in one of the other side rooms listening to my mother's squall: death shoved right up in my face, mocking and pointing a finger.

'Would you like to see him?' the nurse asked. I could read her face; she needed Mum to move. Mum stood unaided, the momentary dramatics over, and she and I followed the nurse into Dad's last room. It was dark, the curtains closed, the air smelling of burnt chocolate. Motionless and mute, his frozen gaze beyond us, Dad looked like he'd left his body while he popped out for a bit. *Angelic*, Sandy said later, *so peaceful*.

We sat by his side, Mum touching his forehead. I touched the back of his large, heavy hands, the ones that used to tickle me and lift me up and rub my shoulders when they ached. They were warm, only his fingertips cooling.

'It was quick,' the nurse said. 'He asked for a drink and then he went.'

'Oh, was it? That's good to know,' Mum said, softly.

I knew that's not what would have happened. He would have drowned in the liquid filling his lungs as his heart failed – a coughing, spluttering, panicked end no doubt. But it would have been quick, she was right about that.

'I'll leave you alone with him,' the nurse said. 'Call if you need anything.'

We watched him for a while, as if something might happen, but he only got colder and less lifelike. It was just the three of us, as it had always been. After a while, Mum and I moved to sit by the window in the half light of the room. There was nothing to do and nowhere to go, the previous melodrama replaced by a weary hush. There he lay – my dad, who had taken me to the garden centre and showed me the stars and picked me up from uni and walked me down the aisle. My dad, who always had a pint of beer in his hand and ugly, practical clothes; who liked eating Stilton and making stir fries and listening to boring talk radio. Soon Mum and I would go home but he wouldn't come with us. He'd go to a cold morgue and lie there alone, and I'd never see him again. I started to cry – stinging tears that made my chest throb.

'I don't want to leave without him.'

Mum turned to me in slow motion, and I gazed up at her, hoping for another arm around my back, a moment of comfort. But her face was different. It wasn't the collapsed wife; the wailing widow; the soft, marshmallowy woman talking to the nurse. It was sharp features and a razor-blade tongue.

'Well, that's the point, isn't it?' she snapped. 'He's dead. He can't come with us.'

My throat went dry, my tears stopped dead on my cheeks. I thought my lungs might burst. There was no kindness for me. Only her grief was allowed.

This moment might have lit the touch paper, and yet it didn't. Our family holiday to America should have nudged me into realisation, or my A-levels result day, or any of the strange conversations we had, but I always ignored the signs and found an excuse for Mum. I told myself that her response this time was because she was grief stricken and, as the widow, her sorrow was bigger than mine. She needed to be cared for, and I should have put my sadness away. It's what any mother in the same position would do. I thought our intense relationship was like that of every other mother and daughter. I had the pieces of the jigsaw, but they were jumbled together with the wrong picture on the front of the box.

As I stood in that hospital side room, I could never have imagined what would happen next. I remember crying at the very thought of Mum one day dying. I believed my perfect mother was my best friend– my closest confidant – and I couldn't imagine living without her. I didn't know that my world was about to shatter and that, in a couple of years, living without her would be what I most desired.

Elinor's Diary

15th November 2008

Rang ward – so so. All to café but ward rang. Alan worse. Raced up stairs and ALAN PASSED AWAY before I got there. I groaned with pain. Helen and I went in to see him looking clean tidy. Still warm. Cried. Brought tea. Questioned nurse who was with him – said his chest was frothy and he said he must eat – and died. Helen took over my mobile and gave it to Peter who phoned Sandy and he brought her. Great comfort. We stayed with him. Then home with Sandy 12pm with his clothes etc. Peter did lunch. Sat and talked and cried. Rang relations – his first then mine. Julia rang – shocked stunned Alan was dead. Had ready meals for tea. Bed slept but 1am Helen and I up talking crying. Then bed with valium and wine.

22nd November

Staggered up – phoned bank. Julia took us. Went to look for hat – no – to bank took 1 hour. Went to Hat shop got hat and scarf. £110 – oh well. Julia fetched us home. Lunch. Rang funeral director – not ready. Finally ready 5:45. V. sad to see Alan in his coffin – Gone. Thanked funeral director. Home via Sainsburys. I did tea. Helen exhausted. 9pm Bed.

Chapter Seventeen

First Scan

We sat in the dingy yellow waiting room of the early pregnancy unit, surrounded by other tense couples, as the nurses skated back and forth. I fanned myself with a magazine while a woman in the seat in front of me swallowed pills that would help her abort her missed miscarriage. The GP had said it was common to bleed, it didn't mean anything and my persistent morning sickness was a good sign. The scan was just a precaution and soon we could tell everyone the good news.

In the stifling semi-darkness of the side room Peter held my hand as I lay on the gurney, a paper sheet tucked into the top of my unbuttoned jeans.

'I'll be quiet for a few minutes so I can concentrate,' the dumpy sonographer said.

Reclining on the gurney, I stared at the ceiling unable to see the screen, the jelly cold on my skin as she pushed the scanner hard onto my stomach. Lying there, it didn't seem so exciting any more. I'd spent all my time envisaging our family and friends' reaction to my pregnancy, but now I was bombarded by 'what if's. I'd had so much reassurance, but there was the tiniest doubt.

'Okay,' said the sonographer, turning to face us and interrupting my thoughts. She didn't turn the screen. 'I'm really sorry to tell you, but I can't find a heartbeat. The size measures six weeks, not eight, which suggests it's bad news…'

I couldn't hear her any more. The darkness was overtaking me. We took the photo home anyway, the small white and grey outline of the baby that wouldn't be. I looked at it once, then hid it away in the back of the filing cabinet. A few days later the cramps started but there were no painkillers on offer, so I stayed at home and spent the early hours of the morning rushing from the bed to the toilet as our baby got flushed away.

And then there were babies everywhere. Everyone we met was pregnant. Adverts were only for formula and nappies. I was surrounded by newborns wherever I went without any hope of having one of my own. My body ached to be pregnant again and I felt furious. There would be no more joy in pregnancy tests or baby scans or midwife appointments. I was a simmering concoction of hormones and resentment.

'There's nothing to prove it existed,' I said, the phone stuck to my face. There had been many phone calls like this over the past fortnight – many moments when I went to Mum, arms outstretched, hoping for some comfort. 'No gravestone, no birth certificate. I wish there was something to show it happened.'

Mum huffed impatiently. 'Well, there isn't,' she said. 'So you just have to get over it.'

It was a jagged meteorite pounding into me. Usually, I'd take her words and swallow them unquestioningly, but this time I'd run out of excuses for her. This time it unleashed a tsunami of fury that rushed over me, unstoppable.

'You wouldn't understand anyway,' I snapped, slamming through my house, the phone burning my face. 'You never wanted a baby. If you'd have had a miscarriage, you wouldn't have been bothered.'

As the last word exited my mouth, I stopped and took a sharp, shocked breath in. I couldn't believe I'd said it. It wasn't untrue; she'd told me relentlessly that she and Dad weren't bothered about having children. But it was Mum's funny story. It wasn't my story to tell. It wasn't meant to be used against her. I heard the intake of air, the dragon ready to roar.

'Yes, I would have,' she retorted. 'You said your body wants to be pregnant again, so that's what would have happened to me.'

She sounded triumphant, as if she was speaking to a naughty child.

'You probably wouldn't have bothered though,' I said, unable to control the wave inside of me. 'The pain it's caused me – physically and emotionally – I don't know whether I want to go through it all again, and I want children.'

'Oh right,' she said, in the same tone she'd used with me when I was a teenager. 'Well, you obviously know best.'

I fumbled to put the receiver in the cradle as our conversation ended, my anger dissolving into a cold sweat of shame. I stared at the phone. How could I have argued with her? She was a brilliant mum, the best under the most awful of circumstances. As she constantly reminded me during my teens, she'd sacrificed her health for me, given me everything she could, protected me from her difficult family. And, ungrateful as I still was, I repaid her with cruelty. I couldn't believe I'd said those things. Shaking, I picked up the phone and redialled.

'Oh hello,' Mum said. My voice was trembling as much as my hands.

'I… I just wanted to call to… to say I'm sorry.'

I felt throttled by the guilt. I was a truly terrible person. What sort of daughter speaks to her mother like that? Mum's pause was loaded.

'I should think so,' she said eventually. 'You've really hurt my feelings. It's not my fault you miscarried.'

'No, I know, I'm sorry.'

'You need to be much kinder to me, Helen.'

'Yes, Mum. I'm sorry.'

She took a slow, deep breath as if considering her next move. 'Well, I'll forgive you this time. But I don't ever want to speak about the miscarriage again.'

'Yes, Mum,' I said, swallowing hard, glass shards cutting into my eyes. 'But do you think it will be okay? Do you think I'll have a baby?'

There was no way of knowing; I knew that. But I desperately craved some reassurance, some hope that I might have the family I wanted, some care from the mother who loved me.

'No, I don't,' she said. 'You'll never be able to carry a baby to full term because your body isn't strong enough.'

I teetered back on my heels and sat on the bottom step, my cheeks burning with humiliation. No, of course not, it was obvious. I couldn't do anything right. I struggled to say the words; they faltered in my tightened throat.

'Yes, Mum.'

Chapter Eighteen

Thin Blue Lines

Mum told me I was no good with children. I'd had little experience; there were no younger siblings or first cousins, only distant relatives whose growing families didn't involve me. I was twelve – a geeky, awkward tween – when I had my first encounter with a baby. I hadn't a clue how to hold an infant, and though I sat on the sofa as instructed, and scooped the warm, soft weight in my arms, the little boy wailed. Perhaps he was hungry, perhaps he was tired, perhaps he wanted his mummy; but I didn't know that, and when Mum used it as evidence to prove my ineptitude, I believed her.

Still, I yearned for my own children. It wasn't broodiness as such, more an innate need to have a family of my own. Maybe it was a desire to redeem the loneliness of my isolated childhood, as I imagined having my own vibrant family, one with siblings and parental involvement and lots of love – everything I hadn't had. I thought Mum wanted that for me too. It would only be natural for my mother to want to see me have my own life, my own children – only natural for her to want to be a grandmother.

It's only now when I look back that I see Mum's meddling attempts to dissuade me. How she sprinkled comments throughout my life, drips of poison, to put me off. *You'll never know guilt like it. You were such a difficult child. It ruins your life. I was so ill during pregnancy. You've no idea what to do with a baby. Your body isn't strong enough to carry to full term.* She must have been so disappointed that, though her comments made me doubt my abilities, I still wanted a baby, even after the miscarriage. I'd understood that I was a failure, that this scheme would come to no good, but her messages had failed to communicate her real point. I wasn't supposed to start my own life, let alone someone else's.

I wanted a baby because I did. There was no reason behind it, no hormonal drive to blame. Nothing was as strong as the desire to try, even if it couldn't work out. So we had sad, resigned sex knowing that a baby could never be.

It was five weeks since the miscarriage when I fixed my eyes on the thin blue lines. I stood in the bathroom and watched them appear, knowing it meant I was pregnant again. I waited for the joy to kick in, that rush of excitement, the smile that couldn't be erased. The seconds ticked past, the clock hands unnervingly loud, but the feelings didn't come. I walked to the mirror and scrutinised my reflection, hoping to recapture the same emotions that I felt the first time, because this was good; this was happy news. I stared at myself, stripped bare of the good and the bad. All I felt was numb.

I've been told that some girls dream of being pregnant like I fantasised about my future wedding. I never imagined floating around in maternity dresses or cradling my bump protectively, so there were no broken dreams when my pregnancy was plagued by sickness. Hyperemesis gravidarum, to give it the official title, wasn't yet popularised by the Duchess of Cambridge's struggles, so my constant nausea, daily vomiting and inability to keep food or water down throughout my pregnancy were referred to as 'extreme morning sickness'. It started a few weeks after I'd taken the test and continued right up until I gave birth, easing only slightly in the third trimester. I tried all the suggested remedies – ginger biscuits, soya milk, drinking before eating – but still ended up in hospital at twelve weeks, a mixture of drugs and water pumped into my dehydrated veins. I remained on anti-sickness medication, terrified I was damaging my baby, throughout the nine months.

The only thing I could find that eased my sickness was rest, and, as I wasn't working, I had ample opportunity. It would take me hours to get out of bed, often only to rush to the loo, having exhausted all attempts to not be sick. I remember that on one visit to the GP to get more tablets, the impatient female doctor haughtily told me that if I went to work, then I probably wouldn't be unwell, as if I were a lazy hypochondriac enjoying each moment of lying in bed with my stomach churning or staring into the toilet bowl. I went home deflated, planning to get up the next day as if I were going to work, but in the morning the sickness rose up in me just the same.

I was ashamed of myself. I was a failure: I didn't work, I was staying in bed. I wanted to be more. I was educated, I was middle class, I was starting a family, but it wasn't enough. I hadn't made a success of work, I wasn't bringing in a second income, I couldn't even do pregnancy well. Funny how I didn't see the parallels between me and Mum, both staying at home, in bed. I felt I was failing her, but I didn't consider that she'd failed me. I wanted to justify myself – prove that I wasn't lazy – but throwing up every day is exhausting; constant nausea is exhausting; being pregnant is exhausting. Why am I giving excuses? I was unwell. I wasn't like my mum.

Elinor's Diary

22nd February 2011
Saw the Doctor – diagnosed Parkinson's Disease – mild, plus dystonia. Home. Rang Sandy, then Helen – shocked. Helen told me off for shocking her. Annette shocked at diagnosis. Told Gwen who said nothing RESULT. Feel terrible – v. shaky all over. Can't stand for long. Rang Judy and Paul to break the news. I said I wanted it all taken away, but would go on till appointment with nurse. Helen had first baby scan. All well, average size.

24th February

Told everyone at church my news. All lovely. Saw Christina told her too. Told all the neighbours – lovely chat. Rang Doris to tell her, left answerphone message – got no response! Cow!

Met Parkinson's nurse – she was wonderful. Says I have typical PD symptoms. Brought home folder. Hairdresser permed my hair which is fine and sparse – suddenly.

Chapter Nineteen

Mild Parkinsonism

Since our conversation about my miscarriage, I'd felt like the earth had cracked: like something seismic had happened, though I couldn't put my finger on it. It wasn't right that Mum hadn't shown concern, instead turning it around to be about her and stabbing me with cruel words. That wasn't what mothers were supposed to do. She'd got away with it before, but this was my grief alone and her lack of care was sharply in focus. Nonetheless, my midwife told me that mothers could act a bit odd when their daughters got pregnant, so I hung on to the hope that once Mum got used to the idea, she might stop being so cruel. Still, it felt like a weak justification.

The sky was a thick, grey canvas as we drove to town in my green Fiesta. I'd resorted to Mum's best-loved activity in the hope that we could salvage a bad weekend together. Conversation had revolved entirely around her new diagnosis. Every time she mentioned it her face lit up, but I longed to talk baby names or ponder the baby's sex or coo over babygrows together. If only Parkinson's Disease wasn't the new favourite.

My bump sat between me and the steering wheel, the seat belt crushing my swollen chest.

'I forgot to tell you,' Mum said, her face breaking into a smile. 'I met up with Judy last week and she was shocked, really shocked, to hear I have Parkinson's.'

My shoulders slumped. Before we'd even arrived at the clothes shop, we were back to the golden child.

'We've been over this, Mum,' I said. 'You don't have Parkinson's. You have mild Parkinsonism. The consultant said it's unlikely to ever turn into full Parkinson's Disease.'

The GP had initially diagnosed her slight shaking of one hand as Benign Essential Tremor, an inherited condition that my Grampy had also had. Nonetheless, Mum insisted on a private neurologist referral with Dr Froome, the local consultant. Even with his more serious diagnosis, Dr Froome said it would be a full decade until the Parkinson's Disease would really affect Mum and, even then it would be manageable with medication. I'd lost count of how many times I'd repeated this to her.

'We'll see,' Mum said. 'Judy was so sympathetic, so kind to me.'

I gripped the steering wheel a little tighter and studied the road ahead. During the past few months Mum had not only refused to tell her friends or our extended family that I was pregnant, but she wanted me to tell them on her behalf. She knew these friends and family members well, spoke to them regularly, and insisted that it was vital they be kept up to date with the news. But she simultaneously dismissed the responsibility to call them as if she couldn't be bothered, as if it was boring to her. Instead I was left to have awkward conversations with acquaintances I hadn't spoken to since my dad's funeral.

'That's funny that you saw Judy,' I ventured. 'You told me it would be strange for you to contact her.'

'She called after you rang her,' Mum said. 'I suggested we meet so I could tell her my news.'

I whipped my head towards her. 'So, you could meet up with Judy to tell her you have mild Parkinsonism, but you couldn't call her to tell her that I was pregnant?'

She threw her hands in the air, her smile dropping. 'What was I supposed to do? Ring all those people up and say, "Hi, I'm just calling to tell you Helen is pregnant"?'

We stopped at the lights and I looked at her. 'That's exactly what you were supposed to do. It's not strange to do that.'

She made a show of rolling her eyes. 'Oh right, well you would know.'

'And they aren't "people",' I said. 'They're your friends. Why did I have to call them?'

She crossed her arms and turned her head away. 'I have had other things going on, you know.'

The light switched to green, and I turned right down the high street. 'I had to explain who I was to Judy. And she thought I was ringing to tell her that you'd died, because the last time I called was when Dad went.'

Mum pulled her hand to her chest, filling the car with her laughter. 'You never told me that.'

I took a sharp breath as I indicated left and parked on the side of the road.

'I don't find that funny,' I said, feeling as if I'd been punched in the chest.

Mum wiped her face. 'You can't park here.'

'I found it very upsetting.'

'There are rules of the road, you know,' she said, pointing at the crossroads several meters in front of me. 'You're not allowed to park here because if you do, someone may die. You'll have to move.'

I unclipped my seatbelt and turned to face her, my bump between us.

'You know, you don't seem interested in me or the baby. All you talk about is the Parkinson's. It's as if you want to be ill.'

She turned away, grasping her navy and gold handbag. 'I can't talk to you about this,' she said, fiddling with the door handle. 'We'll talk another time when I can deal with it. There's the shop I want to go to.'

She swung her legs out of the car before I could say anything more, slamming the door behind her, a huge full stop to the conversation. She crossed the road in front of the car, her shoulders hunched, her worn, black stick leading the way.

Chapter Twenty

Cots

Perusing baby stores is like wandering into a glamorous dream world where having a baby is streamlined and rose tinted. The realities of parenthood have been sterilised – the sleep deprivation, the physical discomfort, the constant contact with poo – and erased in favour of beauty and cleanliness. My best friend, Jemma, and I took turns picking out three-piece suits and tiny, floaty dresses for babies under three months, equally infatuated and incredulous. Jake, Jemma's eighteen-month-old, sat in the pushchair, sucking on a toy while his eyelids fluttered.

'Who would put their baby in this?' Jemma said, holding up an immaculate onesie.

'Why would you dress a baby in white?' I agreed, rubbing my bump. 'It's just asking for trouble.'

'I went to the dentist the other day,' Jemma said. 'It was so exciting, half an hour away from the baby, and you know how I love the dentist. Then they said, "I'm really sorry to tell you, but you've got something on your cardigan." I was covered in baby sick, all down the back of my white cardigan. I really wish they hadn't said anything.'

I was definitely waddling now, my floaty maternity dress resembling a long black tent. I hadn't anticipated May to be so hot.

'Has your Mum told anyone you're pregnant yet?'

'No. But she's told the whole world she's got Parkinson's.'

'She's obsessed,' Jemma said, shaking her head.

I rifled through the sale rack, but it was all spring jackets and cardigans. Jemma was browsing the baby clothes hung up on tiny, wooden coat hangers. She could hide her own pregnant belly, a full six months to go.

'I'm going to look at the furniture,' I said. 'I'll only be a sec.'

I clambered upstairs, relieved to see a rocking chair at the top where I sat to catch my breath. It was even hotter on the second floor, the sun pouring in through the glass-fronted building. It was a relief when my mobile rang, a good excuse to sit a little longer.

'I told Gwen,' Mum said.

'About the baby? That's great news. What did she say?'

I lay back in the chair with a smile. Finally, Mum was joining in with the excitement.

'She said, "What? Eight months pregnant! Why didn't you tell me before?" So I told her all about your miscarriage.'

'Oh, Mum, you didn't,' I said, dropping my head onto my hand.

'Don't worry, she was very sympathetic.'

'I've asked you not to tell anyone,' I said, rubbing my face. 'After you told Sandy I asked you not to, and then when you told Julia I said again.'

Mum tutted. 'What else was I supposed to say? I speak to Gwen every day. I could hardly have said I couldn't be bothered to tell her, could I? I saw Doris on Thursday too and I told her about your miscarriage. Course she had loads of miscarriages before she had her kids. She went very quiet after that.'

I gripped the phone with both hands. I could feel sweat trickling down my neck and between my shoulder blades.

'Of course she did!' I groaned. 'It's not a nice thing to remember.' I slowed my voice, hoping each word would hit its target. 'I've asked you three times now not to tell people. It's private. The news is I'm pregnant, not that I've had a miscarriage.'

There was a thoughtful pause.

'I'm not well, you know,' she said. 'I'm shaking all the time. I've called Sarah, the Parkinson's nurse, and she says she thinks my tablets need changing. I'm going to see her tomorrow.'

I pulled myself up and began to waddle around the showroom. Mum might not be apologising, but the change of subject suggested she'd got the message.

'What are you doing today?' she asked.

'I'm shopping for the baby.'

'Oh,' she said, her disappointment hanging in the air. 'Well, I'll leave you to it.'

Chapter Twenty-One

A Walk

The late spring sun cast a shadow of my swelled stomach onto the tree-lined path as we walked in step with each other. The daffodils had mainly died back, their butter-coloured flowers shrunken and crispy, leaving long patches of teal stems towering above their leaves. I cradled my bump as I walked, the weight pressing down heavily as if the baby might fall out if I didn't hang on. We'd looped the pond once already, but Mum wasn't slowing, the final third of her pale legs striding out beneath her skirt. Maybe it was the sunlight or being outdoors with Mum, but I felt like I did when we were in America.

'I saw the Parkinson's nurse on Monday, and she was wonderful,' Mum said, the light catching her white skin and making her face glow. 'They've put me on a different medication, a stronger one. It's so different. When the doctor told me I had ME, that was it – no further treatment, no doctors involved, off you go and work it out for yourself. But with the Parkinson's I get nurses and consultants and there's so many different drugs and treatments.'

'You don't really mention the ME any more,' I said. She hadn't had a rest that day so her ash-coloured perm was in perfect curls, bobbing around her ears as she walked.

'I still have it.'

'But you do seem much better.'

'Hmm.'

I took an extra step and turned back to her so I could see her face: her smooth peach skin, her baby-blue eyes, her orange-red lipstick.

'This is the furthest I've ever walked with you,' I said. 'It'll be a mile by the time we're home. A few years ago, you couldn't even walk to the corner shop. Don't you think that's amazing?'

She turned away from me as if something had grabbed her attention, but the grassy hill was empty.

'I suppose.'

I laughed and shook my head, brushing my bleached blonde hair from my face. 'I think it's amazing. All those years the ME dominated our lives. All the things you couldn't do – we couldn't do. And now you can walk all this way.'

'Look at those dogs over there,' she said, pointing into the distance.

'I used to pray every night that you'd get better,' I said, refusing to be deterred.

'So did I!' she said, snapping round.

I breathed out a weak laugh. 'I'm surprised you're not happier then?'

She stopped and turned to me, her face shaded in darkness, her back to the dogs. She'd never liked dogs.

'I am happy. But I'm not better. I have three chronic diseases now – ME, Parkinson's and dystonia.'

'That's not what the doctors have said.'

She turned on her heels and strode away, her pace too fast for me and my ballooned belly. She whisked past the playground, taking the hill in large, fast strides as she discarded words in her wake.

'I've been building up to telling you this. You're not going to take it well, I just know.'

I hated it when she spoke to me like this, as if I were an unexploded bomb waiting to go off and she was the innocent victim tiptoeing over eggshells. I was panting to catch her, her voice trailing in the wind.

'I'm getting worse and worse, Helen. I know you don't see it. But I won't be able to come here when the baby is born.'

I stopped at the top of the hill, out of breath. 'What? Why?'

She had stopped several metres ahead, her back towards me. 'You've made it very clear I'm not welcome to stay with you.'

My breath was cold in my lungs. 'That's not what we said. We just want a couple of weeks on our own when the baby is born without anyone staying with us.'

'Alright, alright, you've said it enough times!'

'I've said it once.' I stepped forwards to approach her as if she were a frightened animal, my legs aching beneath me. 'We just want those first weeks on our own.'

'You've made it impossible for me to come,' she said, hands on hips. 'I'm so desperately ill. Until my medication has been sorted there's no way I can come.' She turned and walked away before I could reach her, keeping me firmly behind. 'And anyway, how would I get here?'

'A taxi? Like this time. Or you could ask one of your friends to bring you. You could stay together in a hotel.'

'There's no one who'd be willing to do that.'

'Come on,' I said. 'I could name five of your friends off the top of my head.'

'No, none of them could bring me.'

'Have you asked them?'

'No, but there's no point. I know they couldn't do it.'

I lowered myself onto the next bench, my feet throbbing. I was defeated, unable to persuade her. My head swam – was I being unreasonable? Was it selfish to ask her to stay in a hotel? My friends had done the same when they had their babies, and their parents had been understanding and supportive. And when I'd asked Sandy and Julia, they thought it was a rational decision too. I wanted Mum to be excited, but she was making this so difficult, as if she took no pleasure in her expected grandchild.

'You know what makes me really sad?' I said, shading my eyes. 'Dad would have been thrilled about this baby. He would have gone to the moon and back to get here.'

She reluctantly walked back, stopping in front of the bench, her shadow falling over me. 'I'm going to the moon and back to get to you.'

I shook my head and turned away. 'It doesn't feel like that.' I rested my hands on my belly and rubbed it slowly. The baby was motionless beneath my fingertips, rocked to sleep by the walking.

'Look,' Mum said, sitting down beside me. 'I'll see how this medication goes. See what I can do. I am trying, Helen. But I'm so ill. No one seems to realise how ill I am.'

Elinor's Diary

15th May 2011
Saw Sarah. SHE WAS GREAT PLEASED TO SEE ME
IN FULL TREMOR CONFIRMS DIAGNOSIS AND
DRUG CHANGE. FEEL HAPPIER.

20th May
Spoke to Helen. I am not allowed to stay at Helen's till the 3rd week after the baby is born when I am to look after Helen. SOD THAT. I can stay in hotel. Judy rang – offer to take me to Helen's and stay in hotel for one night.

21st May
Julia and Sandy are shocked I'm being told to stay in hotel and allowed two hours with my family per day. Julia texted later – but strange. Anti-me.

Chapter Twenty-Two

The Cave

I could see them standing at the mouth of the cave silhouetted by the sunlight outside, but they were distant figures. Their voices echoed around me, senseless words that were impossible to understand. Twelve hours earlier, Peter and I had been wandering in the park pondering baby names. As we reached home, the contractions had started – a faint, repressible ache at first – and then my waters had broken.

Lying in a white bed in a white room on the labour suite, I knew Peter was beside me though I could only focus on the intermittent pain. There was a crowd of people around me and someone had said that the baby was stuck.

'Tell us when you have a contraction,' said the petite Indian doctor, standing between my legs. She was grasping hold of something as if ready to pull. It was impossible to follow her instructions, my body and mind entirely disconnected. Time and reality were slippery concepts; there were only periods of pain and then exhaustion in an endlessly repeated cycle. It was a total surprise to me when the baby finally arrived – a red, screaming tangle of legs and arms lumped onto my chest. As I held him, the intensity of the previous hours drained away into throbs throughout my immovable body. There was poking, checking and stitching; two nurses dragging me up into a sitting position; the baby taken away to be checked. Time was no more sensible than when I was in labour. It was only after I'd eaten some cold toast and had a cup of tea that I really saw my baby. Peter had been holding him since he was born, a little bundle wrapped in a towel, his miniature fingers curling around the edge. I held Bailey next to my chest and pored over his screwed-up face. My beautiful, perfect boy.

After we'd told our parents the news – conversations that passed in a blur – I was moved to a quiet side room, the lights low, the walls a clinical pale green. Peter was sent home and, though I was wrecked, Bailey had slept all day and was wired. His first experiences of the world were made as I held him: a vampire-white woman whose hand stung with the cannula, the catheter painless but awkward, lying exhausted and shocked in bed.

Later, when I felt a little stronger, I lifted Bailey into the plastic hospital cot, smoothing his tiny babygrow and tucking the blankets into the sides. His scream was so loud my ears hummed even when he took a breath, and I gawked at him as he spluttered and choked before vomiting thick, black mucus all over his clothes and the blankets. It dribbled down the edges of the cot like tar while I stood by hopelessly.

The midwife was in her fifties with permed hair yellowing at the edges as if she'd been left out in the sun too long.

'Could you help me?'

She crossed her arms. 'You're going to have to do this yourself sooner or later.'

'I don't know where to start.'

Bailey screamed as she stripped him, while I sat on the edge of the bed crying.

'I don't think he likes being in the cot. He's okay when I hold him.'

'Leave him in there,' the midwife instructed as she flew out of the room. 'He'll get used to it. He'll just scream himself to sleep.'

I nodded obediently, knowing there wasn't a chance I would do that to my five-hour-old baby. Instead, I laid him beside me on the bed and I told him the history of the Hundred Years' War. I sang him my favourite songs. I checked my phone, but there was no mobile reception. We both cried. I was very much on my own.

'Now your catheter's been removed you can have breakfast with the other mums,' the midwife said, the electric lights indicating morning though I hadn't slept. I looked at her blankly.

'Come on,' she said, shooing me out of bed. 'Push your baby into the side room and then you can have a nice breakfast.'

The side room was a narrow corridor full of other babies in their plastic hospital cots, all round faced with large eyes and indistinguishable features. I parked Bailey next in the line and examined him, trying to remember something unique. What sort of mother forgets what their baby looks like? In the end I counted – third cot down, second on the right – and nipped into the adjoining room where the other new mums, blanched and bewildered, were scooping unidentifiable hospital food into their mouths. I downed the lumpy porridge with disgust, scooting back to Bailey the moment I'd finished and wheeling him back to the safety of our room. I checked my phone. Another four hours until visiting time and still no mobile reception.

'I've never been so pleased to see anyone,' I said, when Peter arrived.

He kissed my forehead and then Bailey's. 'Home today.'

'They said I might have to stay in another night. I haven't slept. The midwife was horrible.'

'We'll get you home,' he reassured me, smoothing my hair. 'I can take Bailey and you can sleep.'

It was late afternoon when we left the hospital, Bailey curled in his car seat.

'He's perfect,' I said, holding onto Peter a bit too tightly, scared my legs might give way. The car was hot, the sun low in the sky, the day soothingly warm. I lay my head back on the seat while Peter clicked Bailey into the back.

'Have you spoken to Mum?' I asked.

'I messaged her to say I was coming at visiting time.'

'And nothing since? She won't like that. I'd better call her.'

The reassuring hum of the wheels on the tarmac made me feel dozy. The dial tone kept breaking into it, like an early morning alarm interrupting sleep. It rang a little bit too long.

'Hello.' Mum's voice was flat.

'We've just left hospital, we're driving home.'

'Oh.'

'Would you like to come over and meet your new grandson?'

She breathed out heavily. 'No, I don't think so.' There was a long, heavy hollow. 'To be honest, Helen, I don't know why I've come up. I've been here all day, sat on my own in the hotel. You could've at least got one of your friends to text me.'

My chest turned inside out. I should have been looking after her, but I'd abandoned her. I leapt to my defence, a flurry of excuses.

'I haven't been in touch with my friends. I haven't had any mobile signal. I couldn't even contact Peter. We didn't know what was happening. They wanted to keep me in tonight as well.'

'Then you should go home and get some rest,' she snapped. 'Maybe I'll see you tomorrow.'

My voice wheezed out through the tiniest gap in my throat.

'If that's what you want.'

'It is. I'll speak to you tomorrow. Good night.'

My stomach was heavy and sour. I turned the phone over in my hand to find Mum had already cancelled the call. We were close to our house, close to showing Bailey his home for the first time.

'She's not coming over.'

'What?' Peter gasped. I couldn't meet his eye.

'She's angry with me.'

I felt the shame heavy in my stomach. I'd made all the wrong decisions, selfishly prioritising myself rather than caring for Mum. I ought to have let her stay with us; I ought to have made sure she was being cared for; I ought to have put her first.

Peter took a deep breath, exhaling it over the top of the steering wheel before turning back to me and placing a hand on my thigh.

'Call Jemma. Invite her over. She can be the first person to meet Bailey.'

Elinor's Diary

21st July 2011
Maternity is dead area for mobiles so I suggest I wait for call at hotel. I wait and wait and wait. Worried, stressed, angry, upset. Finally call from Helen on way home. She sounds terrible so decide to call off 1st visit and go to dinner. Bad choices. Not nice. Reasonable dinner but all on my own.

22nd July
Met Bailey – lovely. Cuddled him and he liked my Parkin-son's shakes. Cancelled hotel room for tomorrow night and called taxi. Relieved I'm going home.

Chapter Twenty-Three

Jeans

Bailey lay on his play gym staring up with large, curious eyes at the black-and-white patterned octopus that hung from the arches. His legs kicked furiously, strong thighs readying themselves for crawling. Annette sat on the sofa, fidgeting.

'Can I have a cuddle?'

'Of course.'

'Isn't he gorgeous? Just the spit of Peter, isn't he, Ellie?'

Mum met Annette at a toddler group when I was a baby and they'd once been best friends. At some point they'd drifted apart and, from what Mum said, this was directly due to Annette's scepticism about the ME. It was only Mum's diagnosis that had reignited their relationship. Annette's sister had Parkinson's Disease too, and they'd grown closer again as they compared symptoms, exchanged medicinal knowledge and shared a support group. Annette had kindly offered to drive Mum to Nottingham to see Bailey now he was a bit bigger.

Annette was a good shepherd, always coming to the aid of others in their times of need, but she was never a victim herself, downplaying any tragedy or misfortunes of her own as if repelling any suggestion of weakness. When I was a child, Annette had been the dream parent. She was young, cool and energetic in her boyfriend-cut jeans and slogan t-shirts, her spiked hair dyed neon pink: the absolute opposite of Mum.

'How old is he now?' Annette asked.

'Three months.'

'That's gone quick, hasn't it, Ellie?'

Mum sat on the opposite sofa, her floral skirt draped over her crossed legs, which were tanned by her dark tights, her flat, beige shoes pointed in the air. She was staring through Bailey, expressionless and glazed.

'I love babies,' Annette said, powering through the awkwardness. 'Especially one as gorgeous as you.' She tickled Bailey's chin and his laughter burst unexpectedly into the room, a beautiful, abandoned joy.

'Just look how fat he is,' Mum jeered, cutting through our echoed chuckles. Bailey turned to see where the new voice was coming from, his laughter halted. 'I've never seen a baby with thighs as fat as that.'

I took a breath and turned back to Annette. 'Sandy said it's the good milk he's getting. Clotted cream.'

Annette laughed her raucous, machine-gun laugh. 'Absolutely. Your mummy's doing a good job, isn't she?'

'He's huge,' Mum continued, unabated. 'Almost too big for the pram. He's only two months but what size clothes did you say he was in?'

'Three to six months. That's not a bad thing though.'

'You should have seen Helen when she was pregnant. She was enormous.'

'That's comparing her to you,' Annette said. 'You were always skinny.'

Mum uncrossed her legs and turned towards us. 'I didn't look six months pregnant when I was full term. Back in my normal jeans the day after I gave birth. Everyone else on the ward was jealous.'

'I bet they were, love.'

'I didn't eat during my pregnancy though. The midwife told me at one point, "If you don't eat more, this baby won't grow."' Her cackle was hollow, a poor reproduction of Bailey's unbridled glee.

'Do you want a cuddle, Granny?' Annette said, standing and approaching Mum with the baby. Mum's face dropped. She fumbled awkwardly as if unsure how to handle such an item.

'Oh yes. Actually no. I'm feeling really unwell suddenly.'

'Is it time for your meds?' Annette asked. Bailey laid in her arms sucking on a finger.

'I've got about an hour to go. It's always like this.' She held her hands to her face as if she were counting for a game of hide and seek.

'It's alright, love,' Annette said, passing Bailey back to me. He snuggled in, soft and warm against my t-shirt. 'It's probably all the excitement of seeing your family.'

'Maybe,' Mum said, slumping down on the sofa. 'Look at my hand, I'm shaking so much.'

'Why don't you have a drink and relax for a minute.'

Mum shook as she leant forward, an exaggerated display followed by a noisy slurp as she drank her tea.

I wrinkled my nose at Bailey and took him into the kitchen to get a glass of water, his eyes flickering from doorway to ceiling and back to me, adoringly. I stroked his cheek, taking in the velveteen curve beneath my fingertips.

'No, it's no good,' Mum said a little too loudly, making sure that I hadn't escaped her crisis.

'Don't try to walk if you feel that bad,' Annette called, but I could hear Mum's unsteady footsteps approaching.

'I've got to get to my daughter!'

She burst into the kitchen, flinging the door open and throwing herself onto my shoulder. I instinctively moved Bailey away from her.

'I'm so sorry. It's so dreadful, this terrible disease.'

'It's okay, Mum. Do what you need to do.'

'Bye-bye Bailey, beautiful Bailey.' She mimicked a baby wave and then raised her voice in our faces. 'I've got to go, Annette. Can we go?'

'Yes, love, of course.'

Mum staggered to the hallway and Annette led her to the car, Mum's arm threaded through hers. I watched from the doorway, Bailey still in my arms. Once that had been my place beside Mum, guiding her along, keeping her steady. It was a strange mix of jealousy and relief to see myself replaced.

Elinor's Diary

13th May 2012
Took taxi to Helen's, then Peter drove to Center Parcs. Helen told me I'd need a mobility scooter – £51 for 4 days. All tired. To bed.

14th May
Peter restricts my contact with Bailey. To pool – v. crowded. Sat on my own again. Came out – handbag gone!! £35 cash, bank cards, mobile, tablet dispenser and watch. Helen searched and called security. Late afternoon to shop and bought new watch.

15th May
Bad night for Bailey. My pain bad and shaking. Croissants but when I opened oven smoke alarm went off as Peter had put them on rack not tray – but monster daughter screamed at me like a banshee. So shaken I cried. Went to pool again. In PM went for facial with Helen that she'd bought us – quite nice.

Chapter Twenty-Four

Handbag

'Toddlers are knobheads,' Lucy said, plonking Rosa on the floor in front of her.

The toddler group was busy as usual, the baby area crammed with exhausted mothers. We were in a state of disarray, large black crescents beneath our eyes, sagging mum tums hidden beneath loose tops, and nappy bags bulging at the sides beneath our chairs. The children ran around the room choosing between hundreds of primary-coloured toys, the run-down church hall echoing with their laughter and tears, as well as that of their mothers.

'She got her hand stuck down the side of the chair again,' Lucy said, her cheeks flushed with residual anxiety.

'One emergency to another. You've missed a treat,' Jemma said, trying to calm her new baby. 'Anna did a poo explosion so large that even I had to get changed.'

'Hence the attractive nappy-with-a-poncho outfit,' I said, indicating Anna's current attire as she lay in a bouncy chair. 'It was all we could muster up between us.'

'What size is it?' Lucy asked, hardly holding back her laughter.

'It's for a four-year-old,' Jemma said. 'It's exactly the sort of thing I dreamt of dressing my beautiful daughter in.'

Lucy sat wearily on a chair, her t-shirt stretched tight over her bump. She gave Rosa a tight smile as she watched her run off towards the dressing-up clothes. 'What time's coffee?'

'Not soon enough,' I said.

Motherhood is a leveller. It doesn't matter what age you are, what your background is, how much you earn. The babies come and they don't give a monkey's about any of that. They won't sleep, they cry endlessly, they poo all over you and your whole identity from before doesn't matter. We were all clinging on by our fingernails.

Fridays were the golden day. The rest of the week it was just me and Peter. There were no evenings out, no nights away, no breaks. But then there were Fridays. There were other play centres, other toddler groups, but at this one I was cared for. I'd been coming since Bailey was a few months old and, as he approached his first birthday, it had become my weekly highlight.

'Come on then,' Jemma said, stroking Anna's head. 'Tell us about Center Parcs.'

I gave a faux sob. 'Really? We haven't even got wine.'

'It's got to have been better than Christmas,' Lucy said, taking a photo of Rosa in a princess costume.

I laid my head in my hands and looked up at them teasingly. 'Mum's like a child.'

I thought a holiday with my mother was doing the right thing. I thought she'd appreciate being with us. I thought she'd connect with Bailey. I thought, more than anything, I owed it to her. As an only child, there were no siblings to share out the responsibility; the duty fell entirely on me.

Jemma winced. 'Was it exactly the same? Did you have to wait on her all the time?'

'It was worse,' I said, helping Bailey to build a soft brick tower. 'She wouldn't do anything to help out, barely interacted with Bailey. And if she wasn't the centre of attention, then she would storm off, as if she was the baby.' I dropped my head to the side. 'And then she lost her bag.'

The more I thought about it the more I wondered. It was her calm manner as she told us, once we were back at the villa, that she'd left her handbag at the pool. The way she didn't rush back but waited for me to take the initiative. She wasn't going to search the changing rooms; she wasn't going to ask at the help desk; she wasn't going to walk all the way to lost property.

'We went back to the villa after a fruitless hunt,' I said, as Bailey knocked down the tower. 'I asked her what was in the bag and she said a bit of cash – but not her purse with her cards in – her mobile phone – which is ancient – and her watch.'

'That's a bit odd,' Jemma pondered, pulling her hair back from her face in a neat bob. 'Why wasn't her purse there?'

'Quite,' I said. 'But it's the watch that bothers me. My dad gave it to her when I was born. Real sentimental value.'

'Was she upset?' Lucy said, stroking her bump absent-mindedly.

'That's just it,' I said, uncrossing my legs and leaning forward. 'She wasn't bothered. If anything, I'd say she was enjoying all the fuss.'

'Wow,' Jemma said, giving Anna a dummy and bobbing the bouncy chair lightly. 'She's so odd. Did you find it?'

'We searched the villa. I searched her room because I thought she might have hidden it there. But we couldn't find it.'

'Who would steal a bag with a bit of cash, a watch and an old Nokia? You'd just pinch the cash and leave the rest, wouldn't you?' Lucy said.

'That's what I thought,' I said. 'The security people came round. They said the only way someone could dispose of it without them knowing was in the bins. And while they were there, interviewing Mum, she was sort of glowing, enjoying it all.'

Jemma creased her nose. 'That's weird.'

'I could be wrong,' I said. 'But I think she threw it in the bin, caused all the trouble herself.'

'Doesn't sound insane knowing your mum,' Lucy said, checking round the room for Rosa.

'She was so calm about it all,' I continued. 'It was as if she knew exactly where it was. Then she crashed the mobility scooter into the front door of the villa.'

Jemma chortled. 'That couldn't be more attention seeking.'

'I don't know what's wrong with her,' I said, shaking my head. 'There was one point when she had Bailey on her knee – a rare interaction with him – and he wobbled, so she grabbed his face and dug her nail into his cheek – look.'

I pulled my phone out of my bag and flashed the photo, a tear-drop lining Bailey's face in bright angry red. Jemma grasped my phone, pulling a hand over her mouth.

'She's gouged a hole in his face!' Lucy gasped, gawking over Jemma's shoulder. 'What did you do?'

'I sort of covered up for her,' I said. 'I'm so cross with myself. I said it was okay, accidents happen, but what was she doing? She didn't even apologise. We're never going on holiday with her again.'

'You can't have her acting like that. You've got to put Bailey first,' Jemma said.

'And as for the Parkinson's,' I said, making air quotations. 'Her behaviour flits all the time. One minute she'll be telling us she's feeling terrible, she'll have these awful shakes, she needs to go and lie down. And two minutes later she'll bounce out of her room to show us a new dress she's bought. It's bizarre.'

It was unbelievable. I wanted to be sympathetic, but it was clearly exaggerated. The inconsistencies in her behaviour were more than her usual histrionics; whenever the attention wasn't on her, she would create a drama. It forced a visceral reaction in me, a queasiness I couldn't ignore.

Jemma shook her head, 'Have you spoken to any of her friends? She sounds crazy.'

I tutted at myself. 'I don't know whether they'll think I'm being sulky because she's ill and I want her to pay attention to my baby.'

'It doesn't sound like that to me,' Lucy said, helping Rosa into a superhero outfit. 'If you were a bad daughter, you wouldn't have taken her on holiday. And they must have seen some of it too. It's not like she's being subtle.'

'Have you told her you're pregnant?' Jemma asked, and I shook my head.

'We're waiting till Bailey's birthday. I'm dreading it after last time.'

'Oh well,' Jemma said, her smile breaking. 'There's another story I can look forward to hearing.'

A hush had fallen over the room as Cathy strode confidently towards us. In her forties, Cathy dressed as if she were permanently ready to go camping in her three-quarter-length cargo trousers and was the friendliest of the ladies who ran the toddler group.

'Coffee time,' she announced, arms open. 'Would you like me to hold Bailey while you get a drink?' She pulled him up into her arms, where he ogled the patterns on her bubble-hemmed t-shirt. 'I miss them being this small,' she said, smiling at Bailey through her thick-rimmed glasses. 'They're not so cute once they hit their teens.'

I found the three largest mugs of coffee from the mismatched array of cups and balanced the triple chocolate biscuits on top. Jemma and Lucy were in the other room, the one with laminate floor, passing Rosa and Jake sippy cups of squash and pink wafer biscuits.

'Good waitressing skills,' Jemma said, as I passed over the coffee. 'What are you doing this afternoon?'

'Naps all round,' I said. 'And then CBeebies till Daddy gets home.'

She wrapped an arm around me, a gesture that told me that she knew I was putting a good face on.

'Ah, CBeebies,' she said. The children were mashing their food into their faces. 'What would we do without it?'

Chapter Twenty-Five

Julia

The phone rang three times before I hung up, my palms slipping on the receiver. After showering and dressing, I was exhausted; these small mundane tasks were giant obstacles that sapped me of energy. I'd told myself I wouldn't be sick in my second pregnancy, as if somehow I might talk myself out of it. I'd bought stacks of ginger biscuits and healthy snack bars, prepared glasses of soya milk to drink as soon as I woke up, but my good intentions came to nothing. The hyperemesis gravidarum was the same as with my other pregnancies and I'd spent the previous three months fighting endless nausea, my eyes watering as my stomach forced out every last drop of nourishment. I'd started the anti-sickness tablets at six weeks, but I'd still ended up in hospital after a week of failing to keep anything down. While the news reported Kate Middleton's expert care in a private hospital, I spent a few hours alone in a dark side room without a bed as the drugs and rehydration fluid chugged through the cannula in my hand. After a few hours, I was taken to a waiting room in a wheelchair, too weak to walk downstairs. Though I promptly threw up across the floor, I was told by the doctors that there was nothing else they could do.

It was harder during this pregnancy because I had Bailey to care for too and rest was impossible. During the week, caring for Bailey was all on me, no matter how ill I was. So I vomited into nappy bags as I changed him and found plenty of games we could play that allowed me to lie down. Still, he watched too much TV and

I felt horribly guilty. I wanted the best for Bailey, not a mum who needed rests in bed. Not a mum like I'd had.

It was a relief to send him to nursery two mornings a week. It was doing him good, I told myself. He was making friends, having new experiences and I could rest. It wouldn't be for long, just a few months, just until I had the baby and was well again. I was making excuses but feeling like a failure.

Bailey's morning at nursery gave me the opportunity to call Julia though, if I could pluck up the courage to talk to her. I lay back in bed, took three deep breaths and redialled. Julia's voice was soft and melodic, like lying on a cloud. Even back when I was a teenager, she hadn't patronised me. She'd been a safe island, though she was Mum's friend first. She was aged halfway between me and Mum and I'd babysat her children, when they were young, building up a friendship with her of my own. I fumbled to control my voice as she asked how we were, what we'd been doing, if Bailey was sleeping through, finding only mumbled monosyllables to respond.

'I'm calling to ask you something,' I began.

I pictured Julia in her cottage, perhaps sitting in the lounge by the fire, wrapped up in a blanket with her dark ringlets tumbling over her shoulders. Or if it was too warm for a fire, then maybe she was in her little kitchen that overlooked the garden, where she made me tea and comforted me when Dad died.

'I'm wondering if you've noticed Mum acting a bit… strange recently?'

My arms shivered with a cold draught from nowhere. I could feel guilt dripping down from my chest into my sick stomach.

'What do you mean, darling?' Julia said. I swallowed and gave an apology under my breath.

'She's not really interested in anything I tell her about us. I don't think we've talked about anything apart from Parkinson's in months. She seems obsessed. And the doctor said it would never be full Parkinson's, but within twelve months she's complaining of much more severe symptoms. She's always seeing the nurse, getting more medication. And her behaviour is so fluctuating. One minute she's fine, the next she's terrible, and then she pops a pill and *click* she's magically better.'

There was a dazed hush. The voice in my head scolded me for saying too much. I was certain I sounded like I was whinging, as if I thought the world should revolve around me. I listened to every slight movement and the sound of Julia taking a deep breath was like thunder in my ears. She was going to tell me what a bad person I was, how cruel I was being to my suffering, vulnerable mother.

'I have noticed,' she said. The momentary pause gaped wide as I waited for the next sentence. 'I'm so very glad you've called.'

I pulled the duvet up to keep my numb hands from freezing entirely.

'Funnily enough,' she continued, 'I called Sandy the other day to ask her the same question. She thought I was going to tell her off for not taking your Mum's Parkinson's seriously enough. We all feel the same. As you said, it seems to be your Mum's obsession.'

It was like a large glass of water after a long walk. 'You've noticed it too?'

Julia gave a little laugh. 'It's hard not to notice, darling. Her behaviour doesn't match up, does it? The other day I went to see her, and she told me how dreadful she was feeling, how she'd have to go and lie down. But a minute later she came bounding down the stairs to show me a new jumper she'd bought, a completely different woman.'

'Exactly the same happened to us at Center Parcs!'

'And, as you said, she is always going to see the Parkinson's nurse. I'm surprised they don't have a separate line for her.'

I spluttered a laugh. 'She told me the first time she saw the nurse, she gave her a hug. Can you imagine? It's so inappropriate.'

'It really is bizarre,' Julia said. 'Sandy and I have taken her to see the nurse and we've both noticed she visibly brightens and glows when she sees her. It's like she gets joy from having the medical attention.'

'I hear it on the phone too,' I said. 'She'll sound really low and then she'll see the nurse and be bright and happy. I wish I could say it was relief, but it's not like that. She doesn't seem worried about being ill. It's like she's revelling in it. And, have you noticed, she doesn't mention the ME any more?'

'Oh yes,' Julia said. 'It's completely dropped. After all those years—'

'Twenty years!' I blurted, the covers falling down to my waist.

'Twenty years of having ME, and running the ME group, and doing all that internet research and writing the newsletters – and she's dropped it just like that.'

'She says she still has it,' I said. 'But I can't see any signs she does. And when I suggested she was better, she seemed really miffed.'

'We keep reminding her that the consultant said it was mild Parkinsonism. That she's got a good ten years of normal life ahead of her,' Julia said.

'I'm not sure that's what she wants,' I said. 'I think she wants to be ill.'

'She does seem to very much enjoy making a big drama of taking those pills. Sandy and your Mum and I had dinner the other day and she stopped us mid-meal to throw a bit of a wobbly about finding her pills in her bag and taking them very publicly. It does seem to be attention seeking.'

We were talking fast, puzzle pieces falling from the sky as I scrambled to fit them into place.

'I really wish that she would pay some attention to Bailey,' I said. 'But it's all about the Parkinson's.'

Julia murmured in agreement. 'It must be very upsetting, when you have such a precious boy, that she isn't enjoying him as a Granny should.'

When we finished talking, I laid the phone down and threw euphoric punches into the air. I knew later I would feel that flurry of fists beat down into my chest, reminding me of my unacceptable betrayal. But for now, I felt the refreshing relief of not being alone.

Chapter Twenty-Six

Reflection

The website said self-loathing.
It said feeling that you have no right to exist.
It said never feeling good enough and believing you are inherently flawed.
It said feeling powerless and afraid, fearing authority.
It said body issues, either being overweight or afraid of gaining weight.

I'd read a short article in the newspaper about a woman who had cut contact with her mother and I couldn't forget it. Her mother's toxic behaviour was a subtle, psychological abuse that couldn't be easily recorded in a few sentences, but one occasion she wrote about leapt out at me: a peculiar conversation about the author's children that was remarkably similar to the way Mum spoke about Bailey.

The writer had a website and I logged on, curious to read more. It was a labyrinth, a website that I would normally tire of quickly, clicking away when the first pang of frustration kicked in. But even with its bad layout and ever-changing menus, my wet eyes were glued to the screen. Though I would later find other more authoritative websites, this was the first time I saw my experience reflected, the first time I was jolted by recognition that something about my mother wasn't right.

It said constantly questioning yourself, always feeling you make bad decisions.

It said a persistent feeling that the world isn't safe.
It said feeling you're not good enough and a burden to
other people.
It said feeling that you are not worthy of being heard.
It said feeling like you don't deserve to be cared for.

These were my feelings, the indescribable ones that I'd lived with forever. I'd not seen them written down before or heard someone describe them. Reading them made me shudder.

It said that these feelings were typical of children with a
narcissistic parent.
It said that this was caused by emotional abuse.
It said that your parent blamed you, manipulated you,
shamed you.
It said your parent will have insisted you are broken.
It said you're made to feel like you do everything wrong.
It said your parents' bad behaviour is always excused.

It's fashionable now to label someone a narcissist, but the website said a personality disorder is more than egotism or vanity. Narcissistic personality disorder (NPD) is a mental condition which causes people to see the world differently and act in dysfunctional and destructive ways. People with NPD have a distinct lack of empathy and a bloated sense of greatness, viewing themselves and their desires as more important than anything – or anyone – else. They believe they're profoundly special and, to prevent them flying into tantrum-like rages, they need excessive attention to satisfy their self-centred vanity. And they are compulsive liars and skilled manipulators who exploit every relationship for their own gain.

The first time I read the description I couldn't see how my perfect mother fitted. I was blinded, perhaps by denial, subconsciously dismissing the connections and making allowances for Mum's peculiarities and bad behaviour. But there was one sign I couldn't deny. The website said it didn't know why and it didn't know what it meant, but a number of narcissistic parents displayed it.

It said ME.

Chapter Twenty-Seven

Bailey's Birthday

It'd seemed like a good idea at the time to invite Mum to stay for Bailey's first birthday and break the news of my pregnancy to her, but I hadn't thought about the practical implications. My usual afternoon nap was out of the window, exhaustion only intensifying the hyperemesis gravidarum, and I'd spent the day cleaning, interrupted by regular dashes to vomit. I'd collapsed on the sofa just in time for Annette's distinctive silver SUV to park outside our house.

Her car was outdated now, but I could still remember when it was new, looking like a space rocket compared to everyone else's cars. She and her family oozed wealth, and there was no one else I knew who had such brash 1980s money; no one else who had built their own detached house; no one else who had a heated swimming pool; no one else whose annual holidays were spent in a time share abroad.

Dragging myself up, I watched at the window as Annette stood like a chauffeur beside Mum's car door, the slick, black stick appearing first. Annette had once again come to the rescue, driving Mum to Nottingham.

'Your Mum's not feeling well,' Annette said as I opened the door. 'She needs some water straight away to take her pills.'

I filled a glass in the kitchen and held it briefly to my forehead. It could be a blip, I told myself. Mum had been unimpressed when Bailey had taken his first steps, and sulked when one of her birthday presents was a framed image of his footprints, but it was possible that now he was bigger she might enjoy him. Taking a deep breath, I went into the lounge. Mum was sitting on the sofa touching her toes.

'I'll be okay in a minute,' she said, her voice muffled.

'Course you will, love,' Annette said. Her hair was the colour of sour cherries, a pop of chemical pink that glistened next to Mum's usual clothing choices: a beige floral skirt, a white blouse, tawny coloured flats. Mum sat up to receive the glass and gulped down the water before lying back on the sofa and reaching instinctively for the recliner tab.

Annette's shoulders dropped as she lay back on the sofa and turned to me. I noticed she kept a reassuring hand on Mum's back. 'So! How are you?'

'I'm fine—' I began, cut off by a low moan.

'Come on, love,' Annette cooed, drawing soothing circles on Mum's back. 'You'll be okay.'

'This terrible disease,' Mum said, sitting up straight. 'I can't do anything.'

'You've made it all the way here, haven't you?' Annette reassured.

'I've called the nurse every day this week,' Mum said to me. 'And they've increased my medication again. They can't understand it. I'm getting worse and worse, and no one can tell me why.'

'Oh dear,' I said, hoping I sounded convincing. I wanted to sympathise; I really did. But I wished that for once Mum could arrive without the circus. I was far too nauseous to deal with it. 'I think I hear Bailey.'

The nursery was blacked out, the room cool and reviving. I lowered myself into the rocking chair and closed my eyes, listening to Bailey's heavy breathing. It would've been so easy to fall asleep. Was I really that good at covering up how I felt? Mum hadn't noticed how pale I was, though I thought I might faint. I didn't feel like she'd seen me at all. Bailey's thumb popped from his mouth and he sat up. I cuddled him close, his soft warmth against my chest. If I waited for the right amount of time, then Bailey might wake up enough to deal with the visitors, and Mum might complete her crisis. But if I waited too long, I wouldn't be doing my duty towards her. Reluctantly, I got up and carried Bailey downstairs.

'Here I am, Bailey!' Mum announced as we reached the bottom step. 'I've got presents. That'll wake you up.'

I squeezed past her, wrapping Bailey up in my arms. It was too much, too soon. Could she really not remember what it was like to have a small child? Was she really unable to read the room?

'Feeling better?' I asked, taking our usual seat on the sofa.

'Yes, tablet's working now,' she said, dragging a large bag with her as she sat next to me.

'Give him a minute, Mum,' I said as Bailey pulled in closer, his thumb automatically returning to his mouth.

'Look Bailey, chocolate.'

'Mum, no,' I said. 'He's only one. We've talked about this. No chocolate.'

'Your Mummy's so strict, isn't she?' Mum said, drawing her face close to Bailey's while he wriggled away.

'You told me you hated Nanny giving me chocolate,' I said, trying to sound jovial as I moved Bailey to the opposite side. 'Why are you doing the same thing?'

Mum shrugged, leaning back on the sofa and smiling. 'History repeating, I suppose. Anyway, I want to treat him.'

'Give him raisins if you want to treat him.'

She wasn't listening, rifling in her bag and pulling out a train, some pens, a colouring book. She waved them in Bailey's face, ignoring his attempt to climb inside of me to escape the onslaught.

'Ellie, give him a sec. He's sleepy,' Annette said.

Mum shuffled down the sofa, crossing her legs and turning her head away. 'Honestly, I come all this way and he's not even bothered.'

I rubbed my fingers across my forehead and wished she wouldn't make the visit this intense. 'How about I make tea?' I said.

It didn't take long before Bailey was exploring the new toys, rolling the train along the floor and scribbling in the colouring book. Annette sat on the floor, eagerly playing with him while Mum moped on the sofa beside me.

'That's a lovely dress,' she said. I watched her closely. It was the same maxi dress I'd worn the summer I was pregnant with Bailey. 'I don't suppose they do it in my size,' she added.

I suppressed a small smile at the insult. Little did she know.

When Peter came home from work, his face in a taut expression, we went into the garden to admire Bailey's new climbing frame. We all needed the fresh air. Annette and Peter hovered around Bailey as he toddled through the grass, but Mum soon said she was cold, she was tired, she had to sit down, and insisted I took her back inside. While she went upstairs to get a jumper, I stood at the window and watched Peter and Annette in close conversation.

'What was that about?' I asked once Annette had left to go home. Mum was resting upstairs after her busy day while we made dinner. I didn't know if I was hungry or not, the waves of nausea breaking out into gnawing starvation pains before crashing into sickening disgust at the thought of food.

'I was asking her about your mum,' Peter said. 'If she ever found her behaviour odd. You know, the whole ill one moment fine the next.'

I couldn't understand why Annette wasn't picking up on Mum's strange ways, especially when her sister also had Parkinson's. I hadn't felt confident enough to ask her though. Annette seemed to be Mum's most committed supporter and I didn't think she'd open up to me.

'It was interesting,' Peter continued. 'She said that your mum makes such a fuss, you would have thought she was the most severe case at the Parkinson's support group. But she's got the mildest condition there.'

'Did she say anything about the obsession with it? How she doesn't talk to us about anything but Parkinson's?'

He dipped his head. 'She said your mum talks about Bailey a lot at home, but that she knew what we meant. Your mum doesn't show any interest in her either. But she wasn't keen to say much more. Said it will all be fine once your mum gets her meds sorted.'

'Would you like another G&T?' Peter asked Mum at dinner.

I wondered if he could feel the tension in our little dining room, whether he was finding it hard to swallow too. He probably didn't have the churning stomach, the longing to get dinner over with.

'No, I've still got this one,' Mum said, indicating her glass. Peter shrugged and sat down beside the highchair where Bailey was eagerly coating his lips and chin in thick tomato sauce. Mum poked at the pasta with dissatisfaction.

'I haven't told you yet,' I said, trying to repress a nervous grin. 'Bailey's started nursery.'

Mum blew out air, like a deflating balloon. 'I'm so glad,' she said, dropping her fork to her plate. 'You've obviously not been coping. I've been so worried about you.'

I forced a smile. 'It's not because I'm not coping. It's because we're expecting a baby.'

Her face dropped and she gawped at me with dread. 'Bloody hell.'

'Mum!' I gasped, pointing at Bailey.

'Sorry,' she said, letting her face fall into her hands. 'Oh, hell.'

Peter pulled a disgusted face, putting down his own cutlery. 'Do you want that gin now?'

'Yes, quick,' she said, holding her glass heavenward and draining it, repeating the procedure with the second drink.

Peter shook his head and began to clear the table. 'It's good news.'

'I suppose,' Mum said, holding her forehead with a limp hand. Peter clattered the plates into the sink.

'We've had a scan already – would you like to see?' I asked, trying to rid the room of the icy atmosphere.

'Maybe later.'

I couldn't tell if I was upset that she was treating my pregnancy as a tragedy. Or was I amused that she was turning the attention onto herself? I was wrapped in a thick layer of darkness, my feelings numbed.

'No one except Jemma knows,' I said, hoping I might flatter her into a better reaction.

'Thank you for telling me first, at least,' she said, each word dripping with sarcasm. 'You know it'll be a boy. You'll have two boys.' She glowered at me as if she might scare me out of being pregnant.

'Maybe,' I said. 'Which'll be nice for Bailey. Or it might be a girl.'

'Boys are awful,' Mum continued. 'Annette's got four boys and she's told me.'

I stood and wiped Bailey's face gently before picking him up. He toddled off to the living room to play with the trains. In my head this was a statement, a moment of directing Mum's attention to her beautiful grandson, but subtlety wasn't her strong suit.

'Even if they're good when you're out in public, when you're home your life will be a nightmare.'

Bailey was playing with his toys one-handed, sucking his thumb. 'Bailey's not like that though, is he?'

She cocked her head to one side to grab my attention. 'Wait and see.'

Why couldn't she say something better, something normal? She could have leapt around the room with excitement or given me a hug or just said congratulations. Why did it have to be like this? I felt a wave of nausea rise in my throat: not morning sickness, but infuriation.

'I think I need a lie down,' she declared, grasping onto the back of the chair to hoist herself up.

I stood and headed in the opposite direction. 'Do what you need to.'

I listened to her stomping up the stairs like a furious teenager, the weekend ruined for both of us.

'That went well,' Peter said, wrapping his arms around me. 'What a bitch.'

I hushed him, glancing up at the stairs. 'She might hear you.'

'Honestly, I don't care if she does. She was awful.'

'It was probably shock.'

He leaned back to catch my eye. 'All that stuff about boys being terrible? She was trying to upset you.'

It had gone unmentioned for years, but I knew Peter didn't like her. And why should he? She purposefully made a mess so he would have to clear up after her; she gave disapproving looks and tuts; she whispered criticisms of him; she constantly tried to push boundaries. In our first week of marriage she rang him and gave him sex advice, a call Peter and I both tried to forget. And she flirted with him, wilting as she felt his arm muscles, telling him she didn't know what she'd do without him in breathy sighs when he did a practical chore, as if she thought he would be attracted by her weak and helpless act. I should have seen how inappropriate it was, but I was used to swallowing her strange behaviour, however ashamed it made me feel. Every time she visited, instead of confronting the tense atmosphere, I felt torn between the two people I loved the most, unable to make either of them happy. Peter wouldn't accept Mum crossing the line, Mum wouldn't stop trying, and I kept making excuses for her.

'She should be celebrating with us,' he continued, leaning on the counter.

'I'm sure she doesn't mean to upset me,' I said, picking up mugs and stacking them just for something to do. 'She's wound up in her own life. She's not well.'

'She's too ill to say congratulations?'

I dug my hands into my pockets. 'I'm tired,' I said. 'And I feel really sick.'

He wrapped me in his arms again, the warmth of his chest against me, the smell of his familiar aftershave. 'Go and have a rest,' he said. 'I can tidy the mugs.'

Mum and I sat together on our brown leather sofas watching reruns while Peter put Bailey to bed. I'd been counting down the hours until I no longer had to wait on Mum. There had been no more talk of babies. Her bad mood hung in the air and I sat awkwardly, wishing I could say something to defuse her attitude.

'I've been thinking,' Mum said, and I inhaled in preparation of what was to come. 'I'd like to pay for Bailey's nursery fees.'

'Oh.' I sat up straighter and checked myself. 'Thank you. That's kind of you.'

'Well, I can't do any normal grandparent things – babysit or support you physically – because of my health. So it's instead of that.'

'Thank you. You don't have to do that; we understand the situation—'

'I want to,' she said. 'I can easily afford it and it would be my pleasure. I want to be involved, but this illness…' She trailed off and I watched her, the slumped shoulders, her clothes crumpled around her thin, tired body. 'Which reminds me,' she said, suddenly stiffening, 'I don't want a repeat of last time. I was stuck on my own in the hotel all day when you had Bailey, and you didn't even bother to get in touch.'

I was taken off guard.

'I didn't have any mobile reception,' I stumbled. 'I couldn't even contact Peter.' I'd also just had a baby, I hadn't slept in two days and I was completely alone, but adding that felt like it would be too much of an attack on her when she'd just offered to give us £200 a month.

'You've said that before,' she said, her mouth tight. 'But I don't want to be put in that position again. You let me know when the baby's here and I'll see if Annette will bring me again. We'll probably stay overnight and then go. And this time I think I'd better tell the family the news.'

I tensed my jaw. How had we moved so quickly from the kind gesture to be on the attack? She switched seamlessly and I was left flapping in her slipstream.

'I haven't asked you to tell anyone because you weren't keen last time.'

'It took you two days after his birth before you told anyone. It's not polite, Helen,' she said, shaking her head at me.

The backs of my eyes were burning. 'I didn't get home from hospital until Bailey was two days old, Mum. I did it as soon as I could. And anyway, you could have told them.'

'I will this time,' she said, arching her eyebrows as if she were reprimanding an irresponsible child.

'Fine,' I said and tried to regain control of my voice. 'Because last time you refused to tell your friends I was pregnant. You made me call them. And then a few weeks later you rang them all to announce you had Parkinson's.'

The more I thought back on this, the stranger it seemed. She hadn't wanted to tell her friends and relatives the good news about my pregnancy, but she'd delighted in spreading the bad news about her diagnosis. I knew there was something wrong about that, but I wasn't sure why it made me uncomfortable.

'I only called Annette and Judy and Reg and Gwen and Owain and Robin...'

'That's everyone who you should have called to tell I was pregnant!' I chided, crossing my arms. I hated arguing with her, but she was riling me.

'Oh well, I *am* sorry! I've obviously failed you again.'

'No, you haven't,' I said. It was a reflex, a meaningless instinct. I took a measured breath in while my head pounded. I wished I could storm out of the room. I wished I could win the argument. 'I didn't think you'd be interested in telling anyone,' I said, low and defeated. 'But if you'd like to, then that would be great.' I took another breath and tried to change the subject. 'Did I tell you Lucy had her baby? Another little girl.'

'How wonderful!' Mum said, holding a hand to her chest. 'Two girls. The perfect little family.' I closed my eyes. She was too good at this game. 'I would have loved another girl,' she said with a sigh. 'But you were such an awful child.'

'I thought you said I was the perfect child – that I was quiet and good,' I ventured, hoping to catch her out.

'But you didn't eat, and you didn't sleep,' she said. 'I had such trouble with you. Everyone said it was my fault, but of course it wasn't. You were a total nightmare. I kept all your baby things in the loft hoping we'd have another. And if it wasn't for you, then we would have.'

I sucked on my lips. If I hadn't had Bailey, then I would have continued to believe this story. But I knew that babies don't sleep and toddlers are fussy eaters and many people have another baby anyway. Maybe Cathy was right, and Mum had forgotten what it was like to have a little one, but surely baby days should have been rose tinted. For Mum it was like remembering wartime. I only half listened to her as she continued to tell me every terrible crime my baby-self had committed. I knew the stories by heart anyway. No wonder I once believed that having children was the worst thing you could do, but that wasn't my experience at all.

I promise you, I thought, rubbing my belly, *I won't be anything like my mother.*

Chapter Twenty-Eight

Shift

Our lounge was filled with pink cards, piles of washing and primary-coloured toys that engulfed the calm oasis that had been our home pre-children. The sofas we had saved for meticulously were covered in crumbs, speckled milk stains and hastily wiped-up baby sick. Ornaments had been banished to the loft, DVDs raised up a level, leaving only an array of child-friendly items scattered across the floor in a way that I would once have considered unacceptably messy.

Blossom's birth had been an easier experience than Bailey's, partly because I had known what to expect and partly because my head remained clear. After a five-hour labour, I was handed my tiny, red-faced girl with a shock of black hair, her eyes screwed shut, her wild cry echoing in the maternity ward. We took her home a few hours later, Bailey greeting her with a kiss on her forehead, filling my chest with a fizzing warmth that rose like popping candy.

When I'd called Mum with the news, I'd expected her to be thrilled at the arrival of her first granddaughter after the months of negative talk about boys. But her reaction had been flat and underwhelming.

'How much does she weigh?' she asked. I was caught off guard, running on exhausted post-birth adrenaline.

'Don't you want to know her name?' I spluttered.

Though she had given reasons aplenty, Mum's delayed visit was a wordless rebuke for my selfishness when Bailey was born. It was several weeks before she chose to come to Nottingham, and I had to help her organise the trip. I scolded myself for being too hard on her, but it felt like she didn't care about me. Peter's paternity leave had ended, and I was keen to get back to the normal routine of baby groups and play dates. Instead I was trapped at home, waiting by the window, Bailey leaning over the sofa in anticipation of Granny's arrival. I could hear Blossom wriggling in the Moses basket, the same crinkling of wicker which haunted my early mornings, feeling the weight of gathering storm clouds above my head.

'Can you see Granny yet?'

Bailey leaned a little further into the sofa to crane his neck, his darkening blonde hair an untamed mop.

'No… Yes!'

I helped him down to the floor and he ran towards the door. Mum was keen footed from the car, a wave of tequila sunrise lipstick and heavy perfume crashing over us and sweeping through the house.

'Bailey, I've got you a present. Here it is, it's big, hold it carefully, don't drop it! Take it into the living room, there's a good boy. We'll sit here on the floor together. Oh no! I've got my shoes on! Quick, I've got to take them off right now. I've bought some new shoes for wearing in your house, Helen. Where are they? Did we bring in the right bag, Judy? I need the one with the spots on it and the frayed handle. Is it in the car? Oh no, here it is. Do you like them, Helen? They're new. Gorgeous colour, aren't they?'

'Yes, very nice,' I said, backed to the very edge of my living room. 'Bailey, do you want a hand opening that?' His eyes were wide and watery.

'I'll do it,' Mum said, throwing herself towards him, one shoe in her hand. 'Do you like my shoes, Bailey? Red, aren't they? Can you say red? Let's open this parcel. Can you do it? Do you need my help? Here, I'll do it. Too much sticky tape. Oh no, what a terrible Granny I am, putting too much sticky tape on. There we go, open it, open it. It's a toy car.'

Bailey surveyed the car, turning to me with a heavy brow. He hadn't seen Mum in months and this stranger was coming too close, speaking too loudly and with too many words for an eighteen-month-old.

'It's okay,' I said, lowering myself onto the floor and putting my arm around him. He pulled into me, gripping my oversized sweatshirt with one hand and sticking his thumb firmly into his mouth.

'Do you know what it is?' Mum said, ignoring Bailey and pushing on regardless. 'It's a car, brumm brumm.' She took it away from him, driving it around the floor while he blinked at her suspiciously.

'He knows what it is,' I said, trying not to sound short. 'It's just a lot to take in. Would you like some tea?'

'I've spotted Blossom,' Judy said. She'd crept in quietly behind Mum, neatly ordering the abandoned bags in the hallway and standing her high heels next to Mum's caramel loafers. 'Isn't she contented?'

'Would you like a cuddle?'

'No!' Mum shrieked, dropping the car and making Bailey jump. 'You mustn't. You've got to pay the older sibling attention first. I've read all about it.'

'Bailey, would you show Granny your new baby sister?' I suggested.

He pushed himself up, took hold of the edge of the basket and stuck out his chest. 'Baby,' he beamed.

'Oh, so sweet!' Judy said, holding a hand to her heart. She stood at a distance waiting for Mum to approach her grandchildren. Mum teetered forward, like a visitor to the lion enclosure.

'Oh my goodness,' she said, extending her neck to peer into the crib. 'Blossom's face is as long as it is wide.'

Judy turned to me, her mouth wide open and I grimaced in response. I hoped Mum's words spoke for themselves and Judy could see that this wasn't how it should be.

'She's beautiful, Helen,' Judy said, helping me to my feet and then approaching the crib. 'Does she sleep?'

'Yes, she's a brilliant sleeper – for now.'

Judy mock laughed, 'Enjoy it while it lasts. And you, how are you?'

'I need to have a drink,' Mum said before I could reply. 'I'm not feeling well.'

She sat heavily on the sofa and dug down into her handbag, finding a white packet and tossing pills into her mouth. The three of us centred on her as she clung onto the sofa, lying back as if collapsed.

'It just comes over me like this,' she said, since neither Judy nor I had moved. 'Can you see how much I'm shaking? I'm getting worse and worse.'

'I'll get you some water,' I said, taking Bailey's hand and leading him away. I could hear the conversation from the kitchen as I got the glass and turned on the tap.

'Didn't you see the nurse the other day?' Judy asked Mum.

'She's no use. Just got to keep waiting to see if the pills will work. This is the third lot I've tried. None of them seem to do anything for me.'

Mum gulped down the water and took a deep breath. 'Look, there we go. I'm okay now,' she said. I didn't want to be cynical, but the only discernible difference was that her drama had ceased.

'That was quick,' I said.

'Yes, that's what it's like.'

Judy had taken the seat next to Mum. I wondered what was going through her head: whether she saw this as I did, whether she felt confused too. I picked Blossom up and sat on the opposite sofa, letting her melt into the crook of my arm. Bailey had picked up the car and was driving it around the legs of the Moses basket.

'Was it a surprise, to have a granddaughter?' I asked Mum, trying to move the conversation on.

'What? Oh, I suppose so.'

'You thought I'd have another boy, didn't you? That I'd have a boy and even if he was nice in public, my life would be hell at home.'

'I wanted to prepare her,' Mum said, turning with a chuckle to Judy. 'I know what it's like to have boys. Awful.'

Judy had been Mum's friend long enough to know that Mum – with no brothers, sons or nephews – had no knowledge of what boys were like. But I didn't know if she heard Mum like I did.

'Bailey isn't awful,' I said.

'Hmm.'

Her lips were pinched in a sneer and I knew her murmur meant she considered Bailey to be the same as all those boys she apparently knew.

'Wouldn't it have been better to tell me how wonderful life would be with two boys?'

I was pushing her, here in full view, forcing her to confront her own words.

'I suppose so,' she said, through gritted teeth. 'It's just a shame Blossom was born in February. It's such a dark, miserable month. It would have been better to have her in Spring.' I was acutely aware that Mum was born during that perfect time of year.

I took a heavy breath, deflated by the intended criticism. 'I didn't get much choice about that,' I said.

I wanted Mum to be pleased with her new granddaughter – with me – but nothing seemed to be good enough for her. I scolded myself for being too harsh on her; after all, hadn't she tried? She'd brought presents and paid Bailey attention, but it was just so extreme – furious intensity and then cold criticism. I wanted her to walk the middle ground and be the supporting mother who didn't need the attention to be on her. I supposed at least this time I had anticipated what she'd be like and hadn't expected so much.

Bailey cuddled up to me and stroked his sister's head. I turned to look at Mum as Judy took a photo of us. Her face was sour.

Elinor's Diary

10th February 2013
*Took Sandy to Julia's house but OFF period v. bad – shocked
them but ON was so different they were amazed. Same as
at Helen's. Rang Sarah for help.*

10th March
*Rang Sarah – she says this is a bad patch and I will come
through. Saw Consultant. Put me on new additional tablet.*

10th April
*Helen rang to ask me to tell her I was getting confused. We
decided it could be drugs and lack of sleep. Bailey talking so
much better – even phrases. Long to see him and Blossom.
Went to PD Exercise Class, Tai Chi and Self hypnosis. Nearly
60 there. Managed it even without a rest time.*

Chapter Twenty-Nine

Christmas Eve

I glowered at the gold carriage clock that sat on the mantlepiece and watched the minutes disappear. Eighteen years I'd lived in that house, my memories interwoven with the pieces of furniture, unchanged since I'd left home. The decor was a tribute to the late 1970s: the Anaglypta wallpaper that my parents considered timeless had been painted repeatedly in various shades of peach and mis-matched with swirling paisley carpets that they'd deemed to be the epitome of practical yet pleasing. It was as if Mum and Dad had reached a point in their lives from which their tastes and opinions never moved, trapped in the happy memories of their thirties.

It was 11.45 a.m. Mum had been on the computer, playing solitaire, for an hour. I wasn't fanatical about routine, but I knew the consequences of over-hungry toddlers. I'd told her the children needed to eat at midday. I'd told her when we planned Christmas on the phone. I'd told her when we got up that morning. I'd told her half an hour previously.

'I won't be able to do it on my own.'

That's what she'd said when I suggested we have Christmas at her house. I could replay the conversation word for word.

'I know, it's okay. I can help you. We'll do it together.'

The past year had been a chaotic adventure. With two children under two and no family help, it had been, at times, lonely and exhausting. But despite the ever-lengthening to-do list, I'd loved it. The children had brought me to life. Meanwhile, Mum's Parkinson's was quickly worsening despite the consultant's diagnosis. None of the pills worked and her symptoms were increasing in severity. We'd agreed that Christmas would only be manageable if we all mucked in. Nonetheless, I dreaded it. It was a constant compromise and there was no possibility of spending it without Mum since I was the only child.

The clicks on the mouse were infuriating me, like an itch I couldn't reach. I went into the kitchen and noisily searched for the right pan, hoping Mum would come in and decide to help. I searched through the fridge for the ingredients – which I'd ordered online and I'd unpacked. I poured the pasta into the empty pan, boiled the kettle, shoved the bacon under the grill, clattered around – but there was no movement from the computer. The top of my chest was burning. I couldn't believe I was so stupid. I should have known that she'd leave it all to me, like she always did.

I was caught by the smell from the oven behind me. It was unmistakable, the humming in my nostrils that made me want to sneeze. I turned around expecting to see smoke, but instead there were devilish flames licking around the grill. Peter rushed into the kitchen when I shouted, Mum behind him leaping around and flapping her arms. I was stuck to the spot, feeling my blood rushing, fighting the guilt in my veins for supremacy. The fire was tickling the edges of the oven, wild and free and threatening.

'What have you done?' Mum screamed. 'Call the fire brigade!'

Beside me, Peter was calm. He frowned at Mum and took a tea towel from the side.

'Surely we just…'

He closed the oven door and turned off the grill. The fire died away instantly, the charred smell in the air the only evidence. I grabbed his hand, my heart beating hard, sweat pricking on my forehead.

'I don't know what happened,' I said in a whisper.

Peter wrapped an arm around me briefly and then reopened the door. He passed me the tray of still-raw bacon and peered into the oven. 'By the look of it,' he said, pulling a disgusted face, 'it's the layer of grease inside the oven that caused it. It needs a good clean.'

'I don't use the grill!' Mum shrieked. 'And now I won't be able to, will I? You've ruined my oven. I'll have to buy a new one. You've melted all the inside.'

'I didn't know that, did I? I was trying to make lunch for the kids since it's after twelve. I don't know which bit of the oven you don't use. It's not my kitchen.'

I can't remember losing my temper with Mum when I was younger, but recently I'd felt like an unexploded bomb, in danger of blowing up when provoked. I couldn't decide which one of us had become unreasonable.

'Oh, that's right, blame me, it's all my fault,' Mum snapped, turning on her heels and marching out of the room.

'I need to make the lunch!' I called after her. 'The kids need to eat.'

I heard the door to the computer room slam and lock.

Peter shook his head, 'Unbelievable.'

I wiped my forehead and took some deep breaths. My hands were shaking. 'Will it be okay for Christmas dinner?'

'Oh yeah,' he said, wrinkling his nose. 'I mean, don't use the grill again. The rest is fine though.'

'She doesn't need a new one?'

'No,' he said, putting a hand on my shoulder. 'It hasn't damaged it at all. And even if it had, it wasn't your fault.'

Lunch was late.

We sat at the mahogany table, Blossom on the 1980s highchair that had been kept in the loft 'just in case' my parents decided to have another baby. She was rubbing sauce across her bib while Bailey sucked up the pasta happily, picking pleasurably at peas. Mum left the computer desk only when we called her to lunch and nothing more was said about the oven.

'Did I tell you?' she said. 'I went to see the Lilly Fields with Sandy last weekend.'

'You didn't!' I put down my cutlery and gaped at her. She gave a frustrated huff.

'I've told you that I'm struggling, Helen. Over and over I've said it. Running a big house like this isn't easy when you're my age.'

I fought the urge to pick out all the things wrong with her sentence. A three-bed semi was hardly a stately home, Mum was in her sixties, and I was the one who proposed she looked at the retirement complex in the first place. Really it was absurd – she was too young to live there. No one else her age was considering a similar move, but Mum seemed much older than her years and her peers. It wasn't just the drab clothes, the permed hair, the hunched shoulders and the walking stick that created this elderly image. I couldn't remember her being young and fun and active. She had always been old, so it was only right for her to need warden-assisted living in her mid-sixties.

'You told me I was forcing you into a nursing home when I suggested it,' I said.

'Well, I went to look round,' Mum said, closely inspecting her dinner to avoid looking at me. 'And it's nice. I've put my name down. Of course, everyone there is much older than me. But with all my chronic illnesses, I think it will be good. There's help if I need it and those red cord things.'

I shook my head, unable to continue with my dinner.

'They said it could take ages to get a place.'

'That's alright, you're not in a rush, are you?' Peter said, scraping up the last of his meal. Mum murmured in dissatisfied agreement. 'I know,' he continued, 'why don't we take the children in the pushchair this afternoon?'

'That would be fun,' I said. 'I'd love to see inside.'

Mum dropped her knife and fork and the children jumped. 'It's Christmas Eve. They'll never let you in. You have to have a special key. They don't let anyone in.'

Peter laughed at the rush of excuses. 'It's only down the road. If nothing else, we'll have a nice walk.'

Mum's lips were drawn tightly creating a small, disapproving O. 'I'm not coming.'

'I wouldn't expect you to,' I said, returning to my food. 'You'll be going for your rest.'

Mum stabbed a pasta tube aggressively, glowering at me as she chewed, while I fussed over the children and pretended I didn't notice.

She was sitting on the stairs when we got back, as if she'd been waiting for us the whole time, drilling holes through the door with her eyes.

'How was your walk?'

'Good,' said Peter, ignoring the sarcasm, a sleeping Bailey over his shoulder. 'We had a tour of the whole complex.'

Mum folded her arms, towering over us as she stood on the stairs.

'The man on the front desk showed us round,' I said, manoeuvring the pushchair through the door. 'There's so much there – the spa, the hairdresser's, the little shop – it's lovely. And the flats are the perfect size, really manageable. I thought you'd especially like the pool.'

'I wouldn't use the pool.'

'You'd use the jacuzzi.'

'We even saw… Albert, was it?' Peter said.

'Arthur,' I said, 'from the bank. He said it's a great place to live. There's a few people from work there apparently.'

Mum's face was stony. 'Oh. Right.'

'I think you'll be really happy there,' Peter said.

She turned away and walked upstairs without further comment. I met Peter's withering look and knew what he was thinking. That place was too good for her.

Chapter Thirty

A Mark in the Sand

'Oh goodness, are we doing this already?'

Mum was standing in the doorway to the lounge in her polyester floor-length nightie covered with a quilted housecoat. Peter and I had been awake for hours already, feeding the children and trying to keep them from the presents before Mum got up. The Christmas tree was in its usual place in the window, the lights catching the tinsel and sending sparkling illuminations up onto the Artex ceiling.

'Happy Christmas, Granny.'

She groaned. 'I'll have to get a cup of tea first.'

When she returned, she took a seat in the corner, slurping her drink loudly. Peter and I sat on the floor with the children as they dug into the pile of gifts.

'Go and show Granny,' I said to Bailey and he toddled off with a new train.

'Very nice,' she said before he could reach her, lifting her cup as a barrier between them.

'I hope you like these,' I said, handing her three soft parcels.

'Hmm.' It was amazing how little she had to say for me to understand her thoughts completely. 'I can tell who wrapped these,' she said, 'Oh.'

'I got the smallest size I could,' I said as she held aloft the long-sleeved t-shirts she'd asked for.

'I'm far too thin for a size six.'

She was suddenly animated, bouncing on the edge of her chair, sloshing tea as she articulated. 'Everyone's been telling me how the weight is just falling off. Sandy, Annette, Julia. But when I'm with them, I eat well – huge piles of food. I don't know what's wrong, I can't put weight on. Even the doctor's been shocked, but no one can find the problem.'

'You don't eat much fat though, do you?' Peter commented. He was the only one that was showered and dressed, the rest of us mooching in our Christmas pyjamas.

Mum placed down her tea and discarded the presents from her lap. 'I don't eat any fat.'

'That's the problem then,' Peter laughed while Mum scowled.

'I don't like fat. Give me a salad any day, but a cooked breakfast – no thanks.'

'Maybe you need to eat more though,' I said. 'Have full-fat milk, butter on sandwiches, that sort of thing.'

'Why don't you go to the chippy once a week?' Peter said.

'It's all so fatty,' Mum said, her hands on her cheeks.

Peter and I exchanged frustrated looks.

'That's the point, isn't it?' I said.

'If you want to put on weight,' Peter added.

Mum sucked her teeth, slumping back into the chair and picking up her tea again. 'Let's get on with the presents.'

We drove home the following day, the low cloud making the day dark though it was only lunchtime. It was raining a cold, light drizzle that made the air damp. The children were asleep in the back, already forgetting yesterday's Christmas excitement. Blossom's head was laid back, her mouth open, nose in the air. Bailey was sucking his thumb. They were adorable.

'We are never doing that again,' I brooded, as Peter drove. 'She's a nightmare.'

I was wrapped up in my big coat, my hands stuffed between my thighs to keep them warm.

'It was as if we'd gone to serve her,' Peter said. He didn't feel the cold as I did and was dressed in a thin, maroon v-neck and jeans.

He exhaled loudly, his hands anchored on the steering wheel. 'She spent most of the time on that computer.'

'I know,' I said, rubbing my face. 'She didn't even offer to help. It was all moaning about how ill she is, and then – lo and behold – she put the pill to her lips, and she was better again. It's such a joke.'

'Do you think she realises how ridiculous it looks?'

'I think she thinks we'd believe anything,' I said. 'She wants to be ill. She's loving every second of it.'

Outside, winter whizzed past us – the grey road, the clouded sky, the skeletal trees on the verge. It seemed impossible that summer had existed.

'We've got two kids under two, and we're expected to run Christmas from her house without any help. I'm never doing it again.'

I said this without any belief that it would be put into practice. Mum didn't need to drop her voice low and pathetic. She didn't need to remind me I was her only child. She didn't need to list her chronic illnesses. She was my mum. Of course I wasn't going to leave her on her own at Christmas. I loved her.

'I can't believe she's so self-obsessed,' I fumed.

My phone beeped on cue and I let out a moan.

'Listen to this,' I said, '*Hi Helen, how did you find Christmas? Love Mum.*'

Peter chuckled. 'The car must be bugged.'

I leant on my hand. 'What am I supposed to say to that?'

'She obviously knows,' Peter said. 'She's testing you.'

I wrote three different messages before deciding which one to send.

Honestly? Exhausting and stressful.

My heart was beating in my line of sight. I unzipped my coat to cool down and waited for the inevitable ping.

Yes, I thought so.

'She knew!'

'Of course she knew.'

'Not only did she expect us to wait on her, but she knew it was difficult and she didn't offer any help.'

I threw my phone into my handbag and crossed my arms. I wished I could text back something pointed to vent my anger. But I was held back, not only because I could never win, but because I could never do that to her. Part of me felt like I was being unfair.

Peter shook his head. 'She's always been nuts, but you don't think she *does* have a personality disorder, do you?'

'No!' I said, too quickly, too defensively. I took a deep breath. 'No, I don't think so. When I looked at that website, the description didn't fit her.' I rubbed my hands together. 'Why? Do you think she does?'

'I dunno,' he shrugged, 'I don't know enough about it.'

'It's probably just because she lives alone,' I said. 'She's got no one else to think of, so of course she's selfish.'

'I suppose,' Peter said. 'We just have to learn from this.' He put a warm hand onto my leg. 'Take it as a mark in the sand.'

I nodded my agreement fervently. And yet a nagging feeling told me it was more than a little self-absorption. Something about my mother really wasn't right.

Chapter Thirty-One

Reputation

It was Sunday afternoon, and I was chopping vegetables in our large, light kitchen, the roasties in the oven along with the beef, the radio blaring. I finally felt some relief from Mum's strange actions. A corner flat in the Lilly Fields had become available, looking out onto rolling meadows and the railway beyond – perfect. We all knew it would be six months of hell, dealing with solicitors and packing and Mum's moaning, but then, her friends assured me, she'd have a new start. She'd be less stressed, occupied by new friends and activities and have no time to focus on her illnesses. Everything would be better.

Peter came in and turned off the radio, passing me the phone. It was Julia. She said it had happened at church. Mum went to a traditional Anglican church built from light-yellow stone, with large windows and wide pillars which were wrapped in ribbons when there was a wedding. Mum had kept her seat on the dark wooden pews for decades, though she'd swapped the family service for the sparsely populated early Holy Communion once I left home. I didn't know all the older ladies who attended but I could imagine them filling just the first few rows, staring up at the vicar in dewy-eyed reverence.

'She was having a crisis,' Julia said. 'Crying loudly, slumping back on the pew, inconsolable. The ladies were all huddled round her getting her tissues and tea to calm her down. She told them that you're stopping her from going with her chosen estate agent, and that you won't let her pay what she wants for the flat.'

The sting of betrayal stole my breath. I'd spoken to Mum less than twenty-four hours ago and I thought we'd made progress, spoken logically, organised something sensible together. I could replay the conversation word for word.

'This lovely young estate agent came round,' Mum had said, her voice bouncing. 'He told me that I was obviously an old, ill, vulnerable woman who needed to be looked after. So I shook his hand.'

'You can't accept him because you're flattered,' I'd said. It should have been an insult to call her old, ill and vulnerable, but the estate agent seemed to have worked out that for Mum these were the very best compliments. 'What are his percentages? How's he going to advertise your house?'

'Stop it,' she'd snapped, her voice raising. 'You're stressing me out.'

'I'm not trying to upset you. But don't you want the best deal? The best person to sell the house for you?'

'I've shaken his hand now,' she'd muttered.

'It's meaningless. He took advantage. He should know better.'

She'd exhaled heavily. 'Oh, alright. Anyway, I've found out how much they want for the flat, so I have to get that sorted now. It's such a lot of money.'

I'd taken a short nervous breath. 'Aren't you going to haggle?'

'Oh,' she'd said, brightening slightly. 'Yes, I could do that. How much should I start at?'

'I dunno. You're the expert at this, not me,' I'd said. After all, she was the one who had worked on house sales in the bank. She was the one with the career in finance. 'You're in a strong position. Knock ten grand off I guess. As a starting offer.'

'Oh yes, I could do! That sounds much better,' she'd said. 'Yes, I feel good about that.'

She'd sounded happy with my suggestions. There was no hint that she was anything except assertive and ready for the next step. I'd had no idea that she was planning an entirely different next step.

'Why would she do that?' I said to Julia, stumbling back to lean against the wall.

'She was being dramatic, causing a scene like she does so much now,' Julia sighed.

'That's not what I said to her.'

'Of course it wasn't, darling.'

How could she? How could the mum I protected and cared for tell lies about me? There was no way of me restoring my reputation.

'And anyway,' I said, my voice rising. 'What power do I have to stop her doing anything? It's like she's telling people I control her.'

'That's why I thought you ought to know. I'm sorry, darling.'

I put down the phone. I told Peter. I finished making dinner and served it. I helped the children cut up their roast potatoes and scoop up their peas. I put them in bed for their naps. I did it all robotically, as if I was set to serve, and all the time I thought about the people Mum had lied to, who I would never be able to correct. Wasn't I worth more to her than a few minutes' attention?

'Oh hello! What a lovely surprise.'

Mum answered the phone quickly, giddy and breathless as if she had spent the afternoon skipping round the house.

'One of your friends let me know what you were saying at church today,' I said. I was trying to keep my voice level, though inside I was somewhere between furious and terrified. I heard Mum's smile drop.

'Who was it?'

'*Who was it?*' I said, trying to control myself. My words were too well enunciated. 'That's not the point, is it?' I took a deep, steady breath, feeling my heart bouncing around my chest. 'I'm not forcing you to make any decisions. You can do what you want.'

'I can't think of anyone who you'd know who was there.'

'That isn't the point, Mum,' I said, grinding the last word between my teeth. 'You shouldn't have been saying those things.'

'Oh, I know,' she said. 'It was Julia, wasn't it? I should have known she'd be on your side.'

'What do you mean, "*on my side*"?' My emotions were rolling down the hill, gathering speed. 'There aren't sides. I'm not against you. I want you to make good decisions, not waste your money.'

'Hmm,' she said. 'I'll have to be careful what I say in front of Julia in future.'

My words tumbled over each other in my mouth creating frothy noises. 'Maybe you should be careful what you're saying in future,' I said. 'You made me look bad in front of people who don't know me. I'm so upset.'

'Yes,' Mum said. 'I'll be much more careful what I say in future.'

I shook my head violently to try to remove the fog and quickly ended the call. What had happened? This didn't make any sense. My insides felt raw and violated, my head cloudy. Only one thing was clear. My feelings weren't Mum's concern.

Chapter Thirty-Two

The Gap

'Hi Mum, how are you?'

'I saw the Parkinson's nurse yesterday.'

It was a sign that the conversation would be upbeat. I could already tell she was smiling down the phone. Every time she got attention from the nurse she was revived, but when they upped her dose of pills or told her she was getting worse quicker than expected, she was utterly euphoric. There had been no apology for her drama at church, and I would like to have learnt to become more wary of Mum. But things continued as they always had, her illnesses dominating our conversation.

The house was still except for me pulling the washing out of the machine. The children were tucked up in bed for their ever-shortening naps while I did chores. I knew I stood on the cusp of these peaceful hours ending – a time when I could drink a coffee while it was hot and not have to worry about anyone but myself.

'I told her about my accident last week,' Mum said. 'How I fell down the stairs.'

I'd heard this story at least three times and there was an added level of drama with each retelling.

'Did I tell you? I smashed a glass on the floor when I fell and had to crawl to the phone to get the neighbours. They had to use the spare key. I couldn't even make it to the door.'

'Yes, I know,' I said, stepping outside and pegging out some of Blossom's tiny dresses.

'So…' She paused as if expecting a drumroll, the ecstasy in her voice bubbling over. 'They've increased my drugs again. It's made all the difference. I feel like a new woman.'

I hated that I felt so pessimistic, but the cycle was relentless. Mum saw the nurse, she got more drugs, she was happy. But within the week the excitement would ebb away, and the complaints would increase until something dramatic would happen to send her back to the nurse. There was never a breakthrough, no drug that suited her or helped the Parkinson's long term. She was infatuated with getting more pills and being told she was getting worse – not worried, like a hypochondriac, but actively taking pleasure in being unwell. It wasn't normal, but who was I to question it? She was seeing the professionals all the time and they could test her claims of worsening symptoms.

'That's improved things really quickly then,' I said, reaching deeper into the bag of washing.

'Yes,' she said, not hearing my sarcasm. 'But we'll see if it lasts.'

The silence hung between us like the sheets on my washing line so that we could only see each other's shadows.

'Would you like to know how the children are?' I asked.

'Oh,' Mum said, her voice clouding. 'Yes.'

'Only, you haven't asked about them for months.'

When I was in my teens and at uni, it hadn't mattered that Mum was disabled and couldn't do the things normal mums did, because when I needed her she was always at the end of the phone. I needed her now, her support and guidance, her encouragement when I felt inadequate and exhausted. But it seemed her interest in me had run out. She had no joy when the children did something new, no patience to listen when things were hard, no curiosity in what we were doing. She was entirely engrossed in the Parkinson's.

Was I was asking too much? I was a grown up, no longer her responsibility. And yet, I'd heard Lucy and Jemma say that their mums were there for them, picking up the slack and caring when no one else did. Sure, there's a point in everyone's life when roles reverse and the child cares for their parents, but Mum and Dad's decline began when I was seven, and in many ways I'd been parenting my mother since then. Still, I thought that when I had children she would be excited and involved in my life and my family, and I couldn't help but find it suspicious that in the same way the ME had stolen my childhood, the Parkinson's was dominating Bailey and Blossom's. It was like Mum couldn't allow children to come first and steal the attention.

There was a long break, with only the muffled sounds of Mum's cheek brushing against the phone. I waited while she prepared her excuse.

'I don't know if you've noticed, Helen, but I've been very, very ill.'

'I've tried to help, Mum,' I said. 'But you get cross with me. Like with the estate agent. I don't know what to say any more.'

'There's nothing to say, is there?' she snapped. I could hear her walking through the house, picking things up just to put them back down again. 'Anyway, you never tell me anything about the children, so what's the point of me asking?'

The corners of my lips itched. It felt like a sit-com moment waiting to happen.

'I'll tell you anything. What do you want to know?'

'I don't know,' she said, on the back foot. 'How are they?'

'Fine, thanks.'

'See, you don't tell me anything.'

'Sorry. What do you want to know?'

She huffed but I let the gap in conversation hang a while before I spoke. 'Bailey can count to ten now.'

It was a bone, but surely she could do something with it.

'Right.'

The dead air was flat. All the words had been said.

'I'm feeling unwell now thanks to you,' she said. 'I'm going to have to go.'

The phone was dead before I could reply.

I wished I could've felt a sense of victory, proving my point like this, but it only added to my growing despair. Where had my mum gone? I wanted to go back to when we'd spoken daily, to when I thought she was perfect, to when I couldn't imagine my life without my best friend.

I'd come to the conclusion that Mum saw herself as the perpetual victim. She lived in a black and white world, where there were only two possible categories of people: saviour or persecutor. I had been Mum's saviour for many years, working hard to constantly rescue her. But I'd betrayed her by having two little dependants who were using up all my attention and, since I'd abandoned her, then she'd boxed me into the role of persecutor. She could only see me as being controlling, critical and oppressive no matter what I did. I wished I knew how to restore our relationship, but everything I did seemed to widen the gap between us.

Elinor's Diary

14th March 2014
Letter to consultant from Sarah – it says I am getting worse much faster than I should. Feel a lot better today.

15th March
All hell broke loose. The estate agent says they haven't heard from my solicitor. Helen rang and said the obvious. I got cross.

Chapter Thirty-Three

Victim

It's a cliché to say that motherhood is hard. It isn't the work that's difficult, though the banal repetition of childcare sent several of my friends running back, open armed, to paid jobs. Sometimes I felt jealous of their break away from the children, but most of the time I enjoyed organising our days, sandwiching chores between playing with toddlers until I could be enveloped by the peace of nap time. It was the intensity that I found exhausting. The constant to-do list in my head was never reduced because it was interrupted by nappy changes or demands for drinks or snacks, or toys just out of reach. One of the children always needed something and it stripped my mind and memory until I was a blur of a person, rushing to keep all the plates spinning.

I wanted to be a good mum, but what did that look like? I wanted the children to feel love – a knowledge of unconditional acceptance that ran deep in their very beings – something I'd never felt. I wanted them to achieve all they could, reach their potential in a way I hadn't. I wanted them to experience life in all its goodness and never worry or fear or need. And though I tried my best to achieve this, I felt like I was missing the mark. Social media was corrosive, and Jemma and I often mused that the best-looking photos online – the ones where the mum was beaming, the children smiling angelically in clean, ironed and branded clothes, the backdrop hinting at a perfect family day out – probably showed the mum who was falling apart in real life.

It didn't need to be online jiggery pokery though. I was equally outdone by the flawless formula adverts or the perfect parenting on *Topsy and Tim*. I remember reading an article describing what a wonderful, jolly mother Princess Diana had been and doubting that Bailey would describe me as fun and spontaneous in years to come. But then, I didn't have support from family – let alone a nanny – who would deal with some of the day-to-day discipline and domesticity. If I did, then maybe I'd have time to recharge, returning as the exciting, refuelled mum.

I wanted Mum to fit in to our lives. I wanted her to be more than a voice at the end of the phone, but if that was all she could be, then I wanted our conversations to be pleasant and mutual. Mum wasn't interested in our lives though. She didn't want to hear about our days, the successes and achievements or the failures. Her life revolved entirely around her illnesses and we didn't fit into that world. I was calling her less and, though I felt guilty about it, I dreaded her self-obsessed monologues which drained my remaining resources.

Blossom was asleep upstairs, Bailey lying on his stomach commanding the battle of toy soldier-sized *Avengers*. I was going to sound happy to talk to her, I told myself as the phone rang. I hoped it would sound authentic.

'Oh, Helen!' Mum wailed and I knew immediately it was not going be a good chat. 'I'm so glad you've called. I'm absolutely terrible.' I could hear her moving around and imagined her hunched over, grasping onto door frames and the backs of chairs.

'I saw the Parkinson's nurse yesterday and because of that I've had to spend two hours in bed. I can't walk, I can barely lift my head.' Her voice was echoing as she entered the kitchen, her feet scraping on the floor. 'I can't cope with this stress. I'm going to have to call off the house sale.'

'Oh dear,' I said. This was my go-to phrase, uncommitted sympathy that I hated to hear in myself. It wasn't like me; it wasn't who I wanted to be. 'What's happening with the move then?'

The roar began before the words, a rapid crescendo that made me pull the phone away from my ear at its ferocity. 'Don't stress me out!'

I moved into my own kitchen and sat at the table, away from Bailey. I wondered if she could hear the difference in our voices, my soft whisper in response.

'Sorry.'

She didn't miss a beat, her voice switched to a normal volume, pathetic in tone. 'Nothing is happening. The solicitor is dragging his feet.'

'House moves take a long time,' I said, tiptoeing through the conversation in case the lion should return.

'Do they?' she whimpered.

'Of course they do,' I said with a little more confidence. 'You know they do. You remember, at work, all that paperwork and solicitor stuff.'

'The solicitor is useless.'

She was a master in quickly turning from authoritarian to victim, from fury to begging within a sentence. She did it seamlessly, back and forth, building me up and then knocking me down. Yet, in the moment, I never noticed until it was too late.

'If you're not happy, you should tell him,' I said, my voice growing stronger as hers weakened. 'Or if you're really not happy, then maybe you should move solicitor.'

'You don't understand how much stress I'm under,' she said. 'I can't deal with any of it. It's too much.'

Honestly, she was right; I didn't understand. From what she told me she wasn't doing anything. She wasn't decluttering her house, she wasn't contacting the solicitor, she wasn't preparing to move. Instead, she was getting Judy and Annette and Julia to run rings around her while she played martyr.

'I'm only talking about one phone call.'

I should have realised I was walking into a trap. I shouldn't have tried to solve the situation by nudging her to action. I had overstepped the mark.

'You don't get it, do you?' The lion was back, baring its teeth, arching its back.

'One phone call is too much?'

I could hear Blossom crying upstairs. Mum was being unreasonable, and I'd had enough. One phone call, in a day of nothing else, was hardly too much for her.

'Yes.'

'Send me the paperwork and I'll call him then,' I snapped.

'Fine, I will,' she shouted, each word aflame. 'I don't feel well.'

The phone was slammed down like a bomb bursting onto the plain, speeding winds tearing through me and igniting a raging fire inside. She didn't have to deal with any of it; she could just shovel her responsibilities off onto me and repay my diligence with angry phone calls and public lies. She didn't care what I had to deal with as long as she remained the victim.

I fetched Blossom, her face blotchy from crying, and gave her a cuddle. She beamed up at me with those big, baby-blue eyes, her perfect pink lips curling into a smile. I took deep breaths and smiled back at her, trying to calm myself.

'I will never do this to you,' I promised, kissing her soft, round cheeks.

Downstairs, I made the children snacks and drinks, my heart slowly returning to its normal rhythm though the residual panic of how I would manage Mum's house sale lingered at the back of my mind. I really couldn't balance anything more. What on earth was I going to do?

'Can we go to the park, Mummy?' Bailey asked, tipping his head to the side, biscuit crumbs across his mouth.

'Great idea,' I said, wiping his face. 'Let me pack a bag.'

My phone rang as I was popping it into my handbag, a number I didn't recognise. I knelt on the floor and took the call.

'Helen. It's Judy.'

She'd never called me before and her voice was much harsher than usual.

'I've just had a call from your mum in hysterics.'

My shoulders slumped. Again, I was going to have to verbalise something I didn't understand myself. Mum was exaggerating how ill she was for attention and, while I knew there was something dark about her intentions, when I tried to explain to other people, I sounded unreasonable: a spoiled child criticising her vulnerable and lonely mother.

'I know, I've just spoken to her,' I said. Judy had seen what Mum was like. At the very least, she'd witnessed the odd behaviour when they visited Blossom; Elinor's cruel comments, her inexplicable short-lived episodes of illness. I took a breath and prepared to delve into the situation, believing Judy would understand.

'You've really upset her, do you realise?' she said, before I could speak. 'You're causing her so much stress. She says you're making her change solicitor – but she's so ill, she can't deal with that. Don't you know that she's spent the last two days in bed?'

I scoffed, trying to grasp onto something I could challenge. 'That's not what she told me—'

'She's told me that she can't cope with it,' Judy continued. Cutting me off made me sound like an argumentative teenager. I was flustered, but if I could get Judy to listen, then maybe she would understand that things were not what they seemed. The conversation was running away, and I couldn't form the right words.

'She's agreed that I'll deal with the solicitor,' Judy said with finality.

'I suggested to Mum that I take it all over.'

I wanted to justify myself, explain that I wasn't the bad guy. But I knew it sounded like a pathetic excuse.

'No,' Judy said, firmly. 'You need to back off your mother and let me deal with it.'

It was a baseball bat to my chest, a crushing blow. Whatever Mum had told Judy, I knew she'd painted me as a difficult and cruel daughter. I wanted to tell Judy she was being manipulated, but Mum was too good at this game. Her outraged friend – her new saviour – had come to her rescue.

'That's fine with me,' I said, striding into the kitchen, feeling the injustice burn. I said goodbye and stormed around the house, not sure whether I was going to scream or cry. Why had Mum done that to me? I couldn't calm down; my thoughts were ablaze. I took a deep breath and dialled Mum, my head buzzing. She picked up on the second ring.

'Because of you, I won't be able to cook for myself,' she shouted.

I took a swift nasal inhale. 'I'm sorry to have upset you,' I said, chewing on each word and walking quickly upstairs. 'I was trying to help. I did say I'd take on the solicitor if you wanted me to.'

I wanted to sound measured: stern but not tipping into anger. I didn't want her to have anything against me.

'You don't understand how fragile I am. You need to treat me much more gently,' she said, triumphant in her dealings with her persecutor.

'Okay,' I said, going into my bedroom and ripping a cardigan from its hanger. 'Then you need to treat me much more gently. It's extremely upsetting to receive phone calls from your friends as if I was pressurising you to do certain things.'

Mum fell silent.

'Judy called me,' I said, noticing Mum was caught off guard. This was not what she expected to happen, but what had she intended? I pulled the cardigan around me roughly. 'I was feeding the children when she called to say I'm causing you nothing but stress. She says she's taking over the dealings with the solicitor now and I'm to "back off".'

'No,' Mum said. I could hear she was stunned. 'She didn't say that.'

'Oh, yes she did,' I said, going to the window and grasping onto the sill tightly. 'I'm to back off my mother and let Judy deal with it all. So I'm telling you, I won't have anything to do with the house sale any more. I won't speak to you about it. You and Judy can deal with it.'

The hesitation told me that Mum was subdued. She hadn't seen this coming and, for once, the added drama didn't please her. I wondered what was going through her mind, whether there was any regret or protective motherly instinct.

'She really said that?' she said. 'That's not right. I'll have to speak to her.' I imagined her stretching herself up tall to accompany the rising strength in her voice. 'I don't want Judy to deal with the solicitor. I know what I'm doing far more than she does.'

'Whatever,' I said, in an uncharacteristic shrug. 'I won't have phone calls like that again. We're going to the park. I hope you feel better.'

And this time I ended the phone call first. I kept my fingers wrapped tightly around the windowsill and outstared the oak tree opposite my house. I was crumbling, my insides no longer solid, my ankles and knees refusing to support my weight. The floor swallowed me up, the carpet scratching my face as hot tears cascaded. The shaking was uncontrollable, preventing me from going to the children downstairs. It was more than shock, bigger than any emotion I could put a name to: an indescribable breaking of everything I had believed about myself, my life and my mother.

Chapter Thirty-Four

The Box under the Stairs

Mum didn't call or text or email. There was no reconciliation, no explanation, no contact. My emotions had frozen into a large, spiked sphere that sat high inside my chest, fizzing with cold. Every time I moved it jabbed me, reminding me of her betrayal. I couldn't sleep, plagued by nightmares of rejection that seeped into my thoughts during the day: I was unwanted, I was unlovable. I knew Mum was attention seeking, but the episode with Judy was too much. I hadn't realised how little she valued me. I wished that it made a difference to the way I acted towards Mum, but I was never going to stand up to her long term. She expected me to help her sort out her house for the move and we'd arranged for me to stay for the weekend long in advance. As much as I wanted to, I was never going to refuse to go. She was still my mother, and I was still her daughter.

I had driven for three hours through the Friday-night traffic, tightly gripping the steering wheel until my hands ached. I imagined Peter at home giving the children their baths and suppers, reading them stories before bed. I wanted to be with them, not making the long trip to see Mum alone. I knew she'd lied when she told me that she'd cleared the whole house except for my bedroom, but I couldn't back out of my duty. I felt nauseous as I pulled up in front of the yellowy-cream house, taking my bag from the boot in the darkness and wishing I had the guts to turn round and drive home again.

'Oh good, you're here,' Mum said. She opened the door wide, walking into the kitchen without looking at me. The house was worse than I'd expected, the same as it had been at Christmas, piled high with her belongings. Every wall was disguised with furniture; every surface was covered in mounds of paperwork, ornaments, photographs. She was nowhere near ready to move.

'There's a lot to do,' she said, leaning on the kitchen counter, preventing me from fully entering the room. 'You need to finish the loft with Annette tomorrow, there's your bedroom, and all of mine to be done. And you've got to do under the stairs.'

I sagged against the door frame. 'Can I have a drink first?'

'You need to get on with it,' she said, irritably pouring the tea. 'There's a lot to do and not much time to do it.'

'Right,' I said, putting my bag down slowly. 'Let me have a sit down tonight; it was a long journey.'

'You're wasting time,' she snapped, thrusting a scalding teacup into my hands. 'We've got the airing cupboard to do first. All those towels.'

'Can't they go to charity?'

'I don't know which ones you want.'

'I've got my own towels.'

She looked at the ceiling. 'You could have told me.'

I woke at five o'clock in the morning, the cold sphere buzzing, the list of jobs pounding in my mind and making me panic. I dressed quietly in some jeans and a t-shirt and started going through the cupboards in my old room. The house was lifeless, but I was hyper aware, using my old ninja skills so as not to make a sound.

My room was as I had left it fifteen years before. For the first time, it struck me how little it had belonged to me. Though there was a chest of drawers stuffed with juvenile poems and stories, along with my teenage books and stationery, the majority of the furniture belonged to my parents. I'd hated the cream wardrobes which lined the back wall, still full of my parents' photographs and slides. And in the corner, set in contrast to the lilac walls I painted sloppily at fifteen, was a dark mahogany display cabinet with fine china teacups, untouched for decades. As a teenager, I had repeatedly asked for it to be moved elsewhere, but it remained, stubbornly reminding me that the bedroom was not fully mine.

I piled up my childhood, calculating what would fit in my car, listening to the clock tick reassuringly. Two hours passed before I heard Mum pootling downstairs. I longed for coffee and cereal.

'Morning,' I said, carrying a pile of papers into the kitchen. She was standing in an ugly, floor-length, white cotton nightie decorated with small, embroidered flowers, her hair set in curlers. 'Do you have any bin liners?'

'No,' she retorted, putting her hands onto her hips to form sharp triangles.

'No big, black bags?'

'Only plastic bags.'

'Okay,' I said, trying to sound cheery. 'That'll do. I've almost finished in my bedroom. But I've left your photos and ornaments.'

She poured herself some tea, draining the pot pointedly. 'You need to start on my bedroom then.'

I gave a strained smile. 'I'll have a bit of a rest first, maybe some breakfast. I've been up since five.'

'I know,' she said, shakily bringing the cup to her lips. 'You woke me. I tried to get back to sleep but all I could hear was you, rustling papers.'

The spiked sphere started to sting my chest. 'Sorry.'

She pushed past me into the living room, falling into Dad's seat with a heavy sigh, a wordless sign that I was causing her nothing but trouble. I filled up plastic bags with rubbish and recycling, making a mountain that blocked the back door, uncertain where Mum kept her bins. It was eight o'clock and I could hear Mum tapping on the mouse in the study.

'Shall I have some cereal, while you get dressed?'

She didn't respond, keeping her attention planted on the screen. It didn't surprise me that I was expected to do all the work, but I couldn't understand why she was being so thankless. I'd left my kids in order to clear her house and she wasn't even being nice to me. As I boiled the kettle and emptied the teapot of its used bags, Mum's voice echoed from the study.

'I've just remembered…'

I turned and saw her peeking around the corner of the door. It was uncharacteristic for her, hiding away as if she were ashamed to speak.

'I've got to change how much I pay towards the nursery fees.'

'Oh right,' I said. 'In what way?'

Those two mornings a week when Bailey and Blossom went to nursery were bliss. I loved being a mummy, but as we didn't have help from any family, it was an essential break from the intensity of having two toddlers. Mum had generously insisted she paid for both fees, reiterating that this was her way of being involved.

'It's this house move,' Mum said, stepping forwards and leaning a hand onto the wall. 'It costs an awful lot. I need to reduce how much I'm spending.'

'Okay,' I said. 'I did say before that it's okay if you need to lower it, but you said you were alright.'

'Yes. Well. Things have changed.'

Panic was thumping in my chest. Something about this conversation wasn't right.

'How much do you need to reduce it by?'

She took a few steps back so I could only see part of her face. 'Well, all of it.'

'All of it?' I strained my neck to see around the corner. 'And when will the payments finish?'

She was scratching around, her foot circling the floor like an embarrassed child. 'It stopped last month.'

I swallowed. That was an extra £200 I'd have to find for the month. If it was truly because she couldn't afford it, of course I would have understood. But she'd crowed to me about the furniture she was buying for her new flat, the new curtains, the new clothes she continued to buy.

'You could have warned me,' I said, with measured calm. 'That's a lot of money I need to find now.'

'Yes,' she said, and slunk away into the shadows.

I left the kettle to boil alone, rushing upstairs to call Peter. The fear was greater than the fury. How were we going to afford it? But as Peter reassured me, it was the confusion that surfaced. Why hadn't she told me? It had been her boast to our extended family that she paid for the children's mornings at nursery. It was her pleasure – that's what she'd said. So was this punishment? She was cutting herself off from me, cutting herself off from her involvement with her grandchildren. Did she expect me to spit with rage? Or was I supposed to crawl on my knees to her? I didn't feel like doing either of those; I just felt confused, unsure what she wanted from me.

An hour later, when she was finally dressed, she called me to her bedroom. I was being summoned, whistled for like an obedient dog. You can kick it, but it will still come back for more.

The room was unchanged: the scratchy, textured wallpaper, the Ercol furniture, the mirror on top of the wardrobe. I wouldn't be allowed to touch the overflowing drawers or wardrobe full of her clothes, nor the dressing table crammed with decades-old lipsticks and eyeshadows. There was only the blanket box. It was the size of a casket and made of dark, carved wood from an unspecified time long ago, covered in books, papers and a small TV. We carefully removed these items, and began to dig through the photographs, the bedding and the old, crocheted clothing until we reached the bottom of the box. The undulating piles covered Mum's bed.

'What are we going to do with all of this then?' she said, turning to me.

I shook my head. 'I dunno. It's all your stuff. What do you want to do with it?'

'I dunno,' she echoed, her shoulders slouching. 'Let's put it back.'

We heaped the belongings back chaotically. This wasn't my house, these weren't my things and Mum wasn't my responsibility, and that was paralysing both of us.

We were eating lunch when Annette arrived, her neon-pink hair shining with a fresh dye. I wasn't sure if it was their clothes that made them look years apart, Mum in her long, coffee skirt and cream blouse, beside Annette's youthful slogan t-shirt and skinny jeans. Or perhaps it was the way they held themselves: Annette's energy and confidence emanating around the room while Mum sagged against a wall. Either way, it was hard to believe they were the same age.

'Right,' Annette said, wasting no time on formalities. 'Where are the bin bags?'

'Here,' Mum said, hurriedly tiptoeing through her house, hunched over as if in servitude.

'What?' I groaned, my patience finally worn through. 'You said you didn't have any when I asked.'

'I didn't know you meant bin bags,' Mum scoffed, drawing closer to Annette, 'You said bin liners.'

'But that's the same thing!'

Annette stepped forward, stretching out her arms to come between me and Mum. 'Now, now, let's not fight. Come on, we've got a lot of work to do.'

Mum gave a smug smile from behind Annette, and I knew that my reputation as a difficult, controlling daughter preceded me.

'I feel awful,' Mum said, as we reached the landing, touching a limp hand to her forehead.

Annette pulled down the loft ladder while Mum leant heavily on a door frame.

'There you are,' Mum said, as if her work were done. 'Good luck.' She turned on her heels and headed downstairs grasping the banister.

The attic had a certain smell that made me think of adventures and discoveries. Once it had been full of boxes, cairns of books and shadows of possible treasures. Carys and I used to beg my dad to let us explore, balancing precariously on wooden beams and rifling through discarded belongings by the dim orange lights strung from the rafters.

'Oh look,' said Annette, picking up a rusted object that sat on the top of a box. 'Here's Shakespeare's toaster.'

'Why has she kept all this stuff?' I said. 'There's every drawing I did since I was two. And all this baby gear. It's not going to be up to safety standards, is it?'

Annette called downstairs, 'Ellie, what do you want to do with this?'

Mum bounded up the stairs, taking them two at a time and grinning. Annette held the toaster through the hatch and Mum laughed.

'I'd forgotten we even had that. Bin, I suppose?'

'Yes, bin,' Annette said. I could see that this decisive attitude was what Mum had expected from me when we were clearing out the blanket box. She wanted someone else to take control and make the decisions. I heard her heading downstairs again.

'You know,' Annette said, her voice dampened by the dust and darkness. 'It would really help your Mum if you would video call her more often. She's worried the kids will forget her.'

'I *have* tried,' I said, rubbing dust from my jeans. 'But she's not interested. She ignores the children when we call. She only wants to talk about how ill she is. She doesn't even ask how we are.'

'I know,' Annette sympathised. 'She's like that with me too. But once she's moved, it will be different. Life will be better. Just don't stop trying.'

It was easy for Annette to say that, I thought. She was retired with no little children at home, eight hours sleep a night and all the time and energy she wanted to put into trying with Mum. I wondered if she'd had this conversation with Mum too, or whether she considered the maintenance of our relationship to be my responsibility entirely.

It was late afternoon before we descended the ladder, Annette calling Mum up to assess the few bits that weren't broken or rusted.

'I suppose they can go,' Mum said. 'I haven't looked at them in thirty years, so I guess I won't need them for the next few.'

'I'll take these bags to the dump then,' Annette said, leaping up with boundless zest. I didn't know how she continued to sort out Mum's house with such enthusiasm, while Mum played computer games. 'I'll take the charity shop bits next week when I come. Nice to have seen you, Helen.'

I dusted my hands on my filthy trousers as the door closed behind Annette. 'I'm going to have a shower.'

'There's no point, is there? You've got to do the hall cupboard.'

I sat down on the stairs, my legs wobbling beneath me, and glanced up at her. 'What have you been doing while we've been in the loft?'

'I've been on the computer.'

'Right,' I said, crossing my arms. 'Well, I need a break so I'm going to have a shower and go out for a bit.'

'You've come here to help me, Helen,' Mum said, putting her hands on her hips. 'There's a lot to do before you go.'

'You start it,' I said, getting up and squeezing past her. My footsteps were measured so she couldn't accuse me of storming away. 'I'll come and help when I get back.'

'But it's time for my rest,' Mum called behind me. I closed my bedroom door as gently as I could manage. Then I wrapped my hands around my pillow and squeezed it until it choked.

The house was imbued with dread when I came out of the bathroom. I dressed and left the house as quickly and quietly as I could, my legs racing as I walked up the alleyway. It was only then

I could let my pace slow and enjoy the fresh air. The streets were empty as I walked up the hill, the same way I used to walk to school, past Carys's childhood home. Every road had a specific memory, events that were foundational: the church hall where I had Brownies, the park where Carys broke her arm, the statue of an angel in the graveyard that changed position – or so the rumours used to say.

Many of my school friends had been drawn back to our home town as they settled down and began to start their own families. Rachel and Jo had returned, as had Carys who was working at the chemist's adjacent to Mum's doctor's surgery. I spoke infrequently to them all, snatching a drink together when I returned to see Mum. And though Carys's job meant she regularly came into contact with Mum, when Carys and I spoke, I could only graze the surface of what was happening. I couldn't vocalise the situation and was afraid Carys wouldn't believe me. Mum had always been eccentric, and everything I said felt like an inadequate description. It was too big, too complicated, to heave into a light conversation.

I walked through the churchyard towards my primary school, hoping to reminisce in the playground, but times had changed; where it was once an open throughway, there was a locked black gate. I spotted the corner of the school through the bars, but it was no good. Turning back the way I'd come, my shoulders slumped. I really didn't want to go back to Mum's. Instead, I walked along the row of graves near the gates, skim reading the names until I found what I was looking for. After all those years, I knew where it was. I remembered Carys telling me that she had cried until there were no tears left. Her mum, Lynn, had been cruelly stolen by cancer when we were twelve and I cringed at my pathetic teenage efforts to care for Carys as she dealt with her grief and trauma. We were just children, cast adrift, struggling with situations and emotions too large for us. I knelt at Lynn's gravestone and wept. She had been like an aunt to me, but I didn't cry for Carys's mum now. I wept for mine.

None of it seemed to make sense any more. I let my tears stain my face, relieved by their presence, the physical sensation of the hurt inside. Where had my mum gone? I was rejected and humiliated by her, cornered into being her persecutor, when I'd only tried to be a good daughter. How had this happened? If only I knew how to get my mum back, the one who loved me.

I took the longest route back to Mum's, letting my tears air dry, my legs growing heavy the closer I got.

'You need to start sorting the cupboard under the stairs,' Mum said, as I opened the front door. She was bedraggled after her rest, though her orange lipstick had been reapplied.

'I'm really tired,' I said, rubbing my face. 'Can I have a sit down and then I'll do it?'

I peeled off my coat, undid my shoes and flopped on the sofa. It would have been so nice to relive my teens, have a cup of tea together and watch some afternoon telly. We could relax, talk, do something normal. Mum followed me closely and stood over me, blocking the TV.

'You need to get on with it.'

'I will. I just need to sit for five minutes.'

'Well, that's all fine, but there's limited time, Helen.'

I scowled at her, the icy ball spinning inside of me, shards slicing through my chest. She'd spent the day on the computer and in bed, and she was telling me there was limited time. I couldn't hold it in any more, the toxic mix of exhaustion and injustice overruling any patience I had left.

'Fine!' I shouted, leaping up and drawing near to her. 'Come on then!'

I gestured for her to take me to the next assignment, my slave driver cracking the whip. Her Margaret Thatcher-esque assertion dropped; I had conveniently fallen into the persecutor role and she was again the victim. She hunched over, dejectedly looking towards the floor in a pose that made me instinctively ashamed. I followed her to the hall, where she stopped in front of the cupboard and whispered into my ear.

'It's in the back.'

I glared at her, my emotions refusing to be pushed down. 'Why are you whispering?'

'Because people might be listening. What we're going to look at is very valuable.'

I surveyed the hallway with an incredulous frown. 'We're in the middle of the house, Mum. There's no one else here. Who could be listening?'

Mum stroked the wall. 'I think the house has been bugged.'

Paranoia. That was a symptom of Parkinson's. I'd done enough research to know that. She was changed instantly, like she'd peeled off a mask and revealed her insanity.

'Bugged by who?'

'I dunno,' she said, shaking her head.

'I think we're okay, Mum.'

She shrugged and raised her voice to a normal volume. 'Oh, okay.'

I bit my lip, unable to turn away. Was she playing me? Bending down she opened the cupboard while I followed her every move. What was happening? Obediently I followed her instructions, fumbling in the darkness, the dust falling in my hair. I could feel the blunted panic in my chest, a restrained fear of what would happen next. I pulled out hundreds of plastic bags, parts of a long-decayed hoover and finally, right at the back, a large box. I could feel it before I could see it, the frigid metal on my fingertips.

'It's so heavy,' I groaned as I dragged it out by the leather belt looped around it. It was well secured with two locks that appeared to have been untouched for years.

Mum ran her fingers all over. 'I think someone's opened it and stolen stuff.'

'I don't think so, Mum. Look at it. It would be obvious if it had been tampered with.'

'Hmm… I suppose.'

'So, have you got the keys then?'

'Which keys?'

'For the locks.'

'No.'

I took a deep breath in and squeezed my eyes shut. 'Okay. Have you got a pair of scissors to cut the belt?'

'Scissors won't cut through it. You need a saw.'

'Okay,' I said, forcing a smile. 'Have you got a saw?'

'No.'

I stood up and put my hands on my hips. 'What do you want me to do then?'

Mum mirrored me, as if we were on a crime drama, but we were no longer working together. 'I don't know. Put it back I suppose.'

I dropped my head and brushed my hands through my hair. 'Okay then. What's inside it anyway?'

Mum shrugged. 'Some old silver cutlery I think.'

'Cutlery?' I spluttered. 'You think someone's going to try to steal cutlery?'

'It's worth a lot of money,' Mum said, as if I were the crazy one. 'You tidy up, I need to sit down.'

I glanced around the abandoned chaos of the hallway. I needed to leave. I shoved the box, the bags and all the rubbish back into the cupboard as quickly as I could and leaned on it until it clicked. Then I ran upstairs and grabbed my bag.

'I'm off,' I shouted.

'Okay,' Mum said, coming from the computer room, hugging me closely. 'Thanks for coming, it's really lifted that burden. Now your room is sorted, we can have people view the house. I can just potter and do bits and bobs.'

I automatically scanned the rooms I could see. For all my work I'd only scratched the surface. 'I think you'll have to do a bit more than potter.'

'Oh no,' she said. 'The removal men will do the majority when they come.'

'They'll grab it and go, Mum.'

She seemed to grow a foot, standing over me with wide legs, her arms crossed. 'Stop it, Helen. You're stressing me out.'

'Sorry, do it your way,' I said, turning on my heels. 'I've done my bit; the rest is up to you. It's been a huge thing to leave the babies and come here.'

I drove away, my boot clattering with the things I'd decided to keep: a few old toys, an assortment of stationery and a large box bursting with my teenage poems, songs and stories. My scribbled writing was my treasure. I sped down the hill that led towards the motorway, anxiously whipping up the gears and putting my foot down. It was only then that I realised Mum hadn't asked me how I was, how the children were, or anything about us. But her lack of acknowledgement seemed the least of it. I was starting to think Mum was going mad.

Elinor's Diary

25th March 2014
Helen came at 9:30pm last night and went to bed very soon. Helen up at 6am and we had a talk. Then she started on bedroom cupboard. Annette came. In afternoon Helen went to see friends. I made house safer putting away paper piled by door, stuff piled in bathroom. Totally exhausted. She went home in evening dress cos she didn't bring any other clothes like I suggested. House in mess after weekend.

Chapter Thirty-Five

Boundaries

I wanted to enjoy this moment – when the sky was a perfect blue and the sun was bright. I wanted to photograph Mum wearing Bailey's sun hat like a skull cap and know that in years to come we'd laugh at the memory. I wanted to picture Blossom on the same swings that I had played on as a little girl and feel the shimmering heat as history repeated. But none of that was possible. The grief of what should have been was bitter in my mouth.

Mum wasn't pushing Blossom on the swing, she wasn't laughing with Bailey, she wasn't involved at all. And even if she had done those things, it wouldn't have been enough, because it was overshadowed by the lack of memories of her taking me to the park as a child.

'I need to go home,' Mum declared. 'I need to go to bed.'

Yeah. That was more like my childhood memories.

We were lodging in a small B&B, the disaster of the house clearance keeping us from staying with Mum. A large Victorian house, once a manse, it was close to the venue where Carys was getting married, and the owners served delicious homemade breakfast. Though I'd helped the children cut up sausages and bacon, I'd been unable to eat them myself that morning, my stomach churning in anticipation of seeing Mum and the inevitable dramas.

Peter and I sat in the lounge at Mum's after the park, Blossom snoozing on Peter's lap, Bailey fighting sleep as he watched CBeebies. I listened to him rhythmically sucking his thumb, trying to decide if he was dozing without looking at him. Mum was upstairs in bed. It was a relief to be in her house without actually having to be with her, her stranglehold around me loosened while she was resting.

'Mr Tumble's a genius,' Peter said, as we watched TV.

'He really is,' I said. 'He makes it look easy.'

Above the noise of the TV, I heard Mum's footsteps on the stairs, an irregular drumbeat. My stomach dropped; I knew instinctively that her performance was about to begin. I listened, my ears pricked, as she went into the kitchen, waiting for the reassuring sounds of a kettle being turned on or the tap being run, but only Mr Tumble's voice was audible. The folding dining room doors opened, like a stage curtain pulling apart, drawing our attention towards her. Our voices were hushed, even Mr Tumble seemed to fall quiet, all of us focused on the actress. It was clear from that first moment that this play would be a tragedy. Mum's back was bent, her hands were shaking, her footsteps were kept to a minimal shuffle. I knew then that Bailey was awake.

'I'm so unwell!' she wailed, hand to forehead.

Critics might have said that it was clichéd, but the costume department had done a marvel with her wrinkled polyester skirt, ruffled blouse and dishevelled hair. Bailey stared, wide eyed. At three he might not grasp all the subtleties of her act, but he certainly would understand the overall performance. It did not have a U rating; it was not appropriate. Peter hastily called Bailey's attention to the TV and I marched Mum from her stage. She walked upstairs with ease and fell gratefully into bed.

'Why did you get up?' I said, pushing down my fury. 'Why did you come downstairs if you feel this bad?' *In front of Bailey*, I wanted to add. *Why did you do it in front of your little grandson?*

'I wanted you to see how bad I was,' Mum said, her mouth a Cheshire cat smile. Her shaking had been replaced by glee oozing from her pores. The room felt oppressive, as if it were closing in on me, the air heavier and harder to inhale.

'When you feel better, call me,' I said, exiting quickly onto the landing, my skin crawling with invisible ants. I got downstairs and exchanged a silent, incensed look with Peter before going into the kitchen. I stared out at the garden where I had spent my childhood afternoons. It looked dishevelled, overgrown, utterly altered.

'Helen,' I heard Mum call. 'I'm better now. Put the kettle on, I'm coming down.'

I rubbed my arms. *It was almost over*, I told myself. *Only dinner to get through.*

The Beefeater was the sole restaurant I remember eating at with my parents as a child. It was a large, buff square of a building with a veranda that looked out over a car park. It didn't appear to have been updated since the last time I had been there in the mid-1990s, but it was child-friendly. Bailey scribbled furiously in his colouring book while we waited for the food to arrive, blocking out the happy face of a cat with thick, black wax. Blossom sat in her highchair, happily tossing crayons on the floor, studying our reactions.

'What a little madam,' Mum said. 'How are you going to deal with her bad behaviour?'

'She's *one*,' I said, incredulous at both statements. After the post-nap show, I was running low on patience, especially for someone criticising my children. Mum tutted under her breath.

'Ah, here we go,' said Peter, trying to turn the conversation as the waitress arrived with plates full of lasagne, garlic bread, scampi, chicken nuggets and endless bowls of chips. Peter scooped beans onto Blossom's tray, and she picked at them, messily drawing a tomato sauce smile onto her face.

'I don't feel very well,' Mum said. 'I'll have to take my tablets early.'

I knew what that meant. She was a circus master calling the crowds to attend for the matinee performance. She searched in her large, black handbag, the one with a faux gold clasp. The tablets were held aloft to be admired, the golden chalice found, the pills swallowed with visible delight and dismay. I hoped it was enough to keep her desire for attention satisfied, but we'd barely had time to finish our meals, the children still picking at their leftovers.

'It's no good,' Mum said. 'We'll have to go home.'

'Okay,' I said, dropping my head onto my hand. 'I'll take you and come back.'

I couldn't help but feel a little relieved, imagining returning in fifteen minutes and enjoying the rest of the evening with my family. Mum's face fell, her shoulders drooped. I had not given her the right reaction.

'No, no. Actually, I'll be okay. I'll manage.'

Bailey finished his food and returned to his colouring in the most comfortable artistic position, standing on his chair with his bottom in the air, pressing as hard as he could onto the paper.

'Bailey!' Mum hissed across the table, and he stopped, bewildered at the interruption to his art. 'I am going to tell my friends what a badly behaved little boy you are,' she said, staring him down as if to intimidate him into ceasing his colouring.

Peter didn't wait, jumping up from his seat before I had a chance to react, taking Bailey's hand and walking him away to choose an ice cream. I was nailed to the chair, bound fast. Inside me was a battle, my instinct to protect my son fiercely duelling my ingrained duty not to upset my mother.

'I have to go home,' Mum announced, pushing her chair back. 'What?'

'I feel so bad, Helen!' she scolded, her hand back on her forehead. 'But Bailey's having ice cream.'

I wasn't sure if I said it out loud but, before I knew it, we were leaving the restaurant, bundled into the car with Bailey and Blossom crying for dessert. I sat in the front seat, a ball of chained fury.

'Oh, I'm so sorry,' Mum wailed in the back of the car as we drove away, dabbing at invisible tears. 'I wanted this to be the best meal ever, but this terrible, debilitating illness has ruined it.'

The nails came out of me at once, my limbs freed so unexpectedly that it made me jump. The paralysis was replaced by strained muscles trying to hold back my reactions. I turned to her and growled.

'For goodness' sake, don't be so over the top.'

Even the children were silenced.

The car was tense as Peter drove through town, over the round-about and up the hill to my sixth form. A two-minute journey.

'Phew, I'm alright now,' Mum said, leaning forwards. Did she want a cheer? I chewed my lips and bored a hole through the windscreen.

'That's sudden,' said Peter, his voice heavy with sarcasm.

'Yes,' Mum said. 'Well, that's what it's like. An on/off switch.'

I could see her in the rear-view mirror, beaming out of the window, awarding herself five stars for her performance.

'What shall we do now?' she said.

Did she really not understand what she'd done?

'We're taking you home,' Peter said, before I could respond, and Mum's smile dropped. She was expecting flowers to be thrown, calls for an encore, at the very least a lengthy applause. That was how it had been for her in the past; she made a dramatic scene and people came running. But it didn't work when she made it so obvious it was exaggerated.

We parked outside her house and I opened the car door for her. She got out and walked up her drive without acknowledging me. I followed at a distance.

'Oh, there you are,' she said, turning towards me as she unlocked her front door. 'I thought you'd disappeared.'

I scowled. 'Disappeared where?'

She wrapped her arms around me, as a performer at the end of the show. 'Don't worry about me, Helen. I'll be okay. You mustn't worry.'

Had she been witnessing the same events I had? Or was she somewhere else entirely? She closed the door behind her before I could say anything that might taint the moment, retiring in the afterglow of her performance. I walked back to the car, my vision blurred, my mind spinning. I crossed my arms to subdue my shaking.

'We are never having dinner with my mother again.'

Chapter Thirty-Six

Vertigo

The pushchair pulled me along, my feet floating above the pavement as I headed towards the Friday toddler group. I was swaying out of control, unable to touch solid ground, the children's chatter a background noise.

The website about parents with NPD had planted a tiny seed of doubt that had burrowed down into my mind and sprouted with every encounter I'd had with my mother. Though I'd shrugged it off before, ignored the nagging concerns, now I returned to the website I could see how closely Mum fitted the profile.

> It said narcissistic parents need to be the centre of attention.
> It said they revel in creating dramas.
> It said they enjoy other people's failures.
> It said they lack empathy.
> It said they exaggerate.
> It said they lie about everything.
> It said they are constantly the victim.
> It said they are vain.
> It said they resent other people's successes.
> It said they fake illnesses.
> It said they manipulate for their own gain.
> It said their descriptions of the past can't be trusted.
> It said ME.

The more I read, the more I realised a striking symptom of Mum's NPD was the faking of illnesses, or Munchausen's Syndrome. I became an armchair researcher, skipping through online articles about a disorder where people deceive their family, friends and doctors by falsifying symptoms, injuring themselves, consuming drugs they don't need or altering laboratory samples. A mental illness dressed up as a physical one, people with Munchausen's know they're pretending to be unwell, but their gain isn't financial or material. Rather, playing 'the sick person' gives them sympathy, attention and a valuable place in society. Often a symptom of a personality disorder, such as narcissism, Munchausen's is rarely detected since patients go to extreme lengths to convince medical professionals and choose symptoms that are hard to disprove, such as headaches, seizures and fainting fits.

Mum couldn't have faked ME for twenty years, could she? She couldn't have lied for that long to me and my dad, to her friends, to our wider family. She wouldn't have sat on the ME group committee, run the meetings, been the treasurer, written the newsletters for years, when she didn't really have ME. She wasn't cruel enough to have mocked us all.

Unless faking an illness got Mum the attention she desired and being disabled gave her endless sympathy from friends, family and strangers. She'd used a stick to walk. She'd gone shopping in an electric wheelchair. ME might be an invisible illness, but Mum made it conspicuous. No one else knew as much about ME as she did – she was the local expert. As secretary and treasurer for the ME group, she had success and praise. She'd even been presented with a certificate that hailed her as a 'Local Health Champion', the local papers printing a list of her achievements alongside her beaming photo. Her ME work had doubled her identity as victim; not only was she unwell, but she was also using all of her limited energy to serve others. And though her 'disability' meant that Dad and I had sacrificed our hopes and desires, she was getting more and more attention. Could it really be that my whole childhood experience had been founded on a lie?

The world was hazy, whirling around me as if I'd come off the Waltzers. My cold, white fingers were wrapped around the pushchair as I entered the church hall.

'Are you alright?' Jemma asked, coming up to me as I stood in the queue to pay. She was a blur.

'No,' I said, too numb to cry. She took my arm and sat me down in the baby area, though our little ones were too big for it now. Together we unclipped Bailey and Blossom from the pushchair and let them run away to play.

'I called Mum's friends,' I explained, in our moment of childless-ness. 'They've known her for years. I wanted to know if it was in my head.'

'Or in your Mum's,' Jemma said, and I spluttered a laugh. 'What did they say?'

'Julia said she knew Mum was a manipulative person from the moment she met her,' I confided. 'And Sandy told me that they used to go on shopping trips while I was at school. Mum would spend hours and hours on her feet shopping for clothes. All day she'd be going and never once have to sit down or take a rest.'

'Oh my life,' Jemma said, grasping my hand. 'When she couldn't walk down the road with you.'

'Exactly,' I said, my voice a monotone. 'And Sandy said that loads of people used to question whether Mum's ME was real. But Mum was her friend, so she believed her.'

'Of course she did,' Jemma said. 'You don't expect people to lie about something like that.'

'It was my life,' I said. 'I was the daughter of two disabled parents – but it wasn't true. All those things I did for her or didn't do because of her. I feel so stupid.'

Jemma wrapped her arms around me. 'You are not stupid at all. You are wonderful and caring and she took advantage of that.'

I leant on Jemma's shoulder, feeling like a dead weight. 'It's so big, you know?'

'Huge,' she said, pulling back and examining my dry face. 'I can't imagine how you must be feeling.'

'Dizzy,' I said. 'I don't know who to trust. I keep thinking this is me being a horrible daughter but then I remember what she's been doing.'

'She's definitely the horrible one,' Jemma said, 'But what do you do with that? She's still your mum.' I nodded wearily as Jemma stood up, spying over the crowd of children. 'Hold on, someone's stolen Anna's doll and she looks like she might wallop them.'

I laughed, rubbing my face as Jemma trotted away to intervene. I didn't know what to do with the information I had gathered. The way things were between us, I couldn't face Mum with the accusation of her faking the ME. I feared she might end our relationship entirely. She'd distanced herself from relatives and friends who had doubted her before, and all I had were opinions and speculations with no idea where Julia and Sandy's interests were vested. Mum had told me repeatedly over the years that news corporations, the government and the NHS were all set against ME, as if it were some Area 51 secret. The same could be true of normal people with their own egos and selfish desires. Truth was like water, sliding through my fingers, thirst-quenching relief out of reach.

I checked my face in the plastic mirror attached to the pushchair and, reassured that I looked vaguely normal, I went to the counter to pay my one-pound entry. Cathy was holding Lucy's new baby.

'I was asking around if anyone would mind leading the singing this week. Our usual lady's away,' Cathy said.

'I definitely won't,' Lucy said, taking the baby back. 'I hate being up in front of everyone.'

I examined Lucy's cheek, unable to turn away. Her words were bumping up against the wall of my mind, incapable of entering. They repeated in my head: she didn't want to do it, so she wasn't going to. I wanted to laugh, but I knew it would come out as a frenzied, psychotic cackle. I'd had disabled parents, so I'd had to do things I didn't want to do. I'd had to do things I wasn't ready for, things I wasn't able to do properly because I was too young. My choices had been irrelevant because my parents couldn't do those things. Unless, of course, Mum could do them, but decided not to, in which case I'd spent most of my life forfeiting my needs for a lie.

Cathy was pulling me into the kitchen, my vacant eyes flicking through the toddler group, my face burning. It was the first time I'd been there, in the small back room amongst the 1980s counters and the two huge identical ovens.

'Are you okay?' she asked, keeping a reassuring hand on my shoulder. She had a zipped hoodie on today over a floaty blouse and her usual cropped, beige camping trousers.

'I'm fine,' I replied automatically..

'What's happened?'

I told her about the wedding weekend, Mum's paranoia during the house clearing, the website, the reactions of her friends…

If I'd been thinking straight, then I'd have heard the unusual coolness in Cathy's voice as she responded with monosyllables. I would have noticed that she'd stepped back from me, removing her comforting hands and heaving them onto her hips. I would have realised Cathy didn't understand.

'It's obvious Mum's exaggerating the Parkinson's. But now I'm starting to think she didn't have ME either. It was all a big lie. My whole childhood was based on a lie. The story of my life was that I had disabled parents. But that was a lie. Everything was built on a lie.'

The words were tumbling out in dry sobs that I couldn't stop. Everything was swirling and I wanted to sit down.

'No. It wasn't a lie,' Cathy said, as if she was giving me an unquestionable fact. 'It's a different point of view. Like if I went out for the day with my parents when I was a child and had a wonderful day, but they had a horrible day. It doesn't mean it wasn't a good day for me.'

'No, no. It's bigger than that.' I shook my head, fumbling for words, unable to argue because there was no longer truth or logic. 'It's not perspective. She wasn't ill. My dad and I based our whole lives around her being ill and it wasn't true. She was pretending. I thought she was my best friend. But she was lying to me. She's always lied to me.'

'No,' Cathy continued. 'She *was* your best friend. Whether or not she had ME doesn't change anything. She's your mum.' She sighed heavily. 'You've got to stop saying you've been abused.'

I recoiled, examining her face, as if she were a stranger. She'd been so kind to me before and I couldn't understand what had changed.

'I've never said I was abused.'

Cathy picked up a cloth and began scrubbing the surfaces. 'I've seen abuse. I've seen those families close up in my job. You know,' she said, shaking her head, 'you're acting like my sister. She says we had a bad childhood because our parents made us eat everything on our plates before we left the table. But it's hardly abuse, is it?'

Her words were pummelling me. I didn't understand why she was being so adamant, so unwilling to hear me. Did she think she was being comforting, or helpful? I felt like she was saying I was the problem; I was the bad daughter; I was failing my mother again.

I began to back away towards the door, grasping onto the counters to steady myself and hoping that, somehow, I'd find my way back to Jemma. The tears were pouring down my face, some dripping onto my t-shirt, some marking the floor.

'You've got to stop focusing on the bad times and think about the good things. Your mum's obviously finding things hard at the moment, but you've got to care for her like she's cared for you. She's your mum, Helen. You've got to stop acting like this.'

I ended the conversation quickly and stepped out of the kitchen, gathering Bailey and Blossom with as few words as I could. I shook my head at Jemma, and she nodded in acknowledgement that I couldn't talk. Holding her fingers to her ear she signalled she would call later. I didn't even care if I had all my things, I needed to get out.

I was home in a few steps without any recollection of the walk. My mind was whirring – a nauseous mix of self-doubt and anger. I'd never said I was abused. I wasn't like Cathy's sister. But Cathy was my friend so I couldn't help but doubt myself. I dug through my memories, desperately searching for something good to remember, some gloriously technicoloured moment that would prove I wasn't focusing on the bad. But the negatives were irreparable. Everything was tainted by Mum's lie.

My temples were pounding, my sight smudged and clouded. What Cathy didn't seem to understand was that Mum hadn't told an insignificant one-off, inconsequential fib. Her lie had spanned decades and it changed everything. Her ME had shaped my whole life, all my experiences and who I'd become, and it was no less of a deception because she was my mother.

I was crumbling. What sort of mother lies and makes life worse than it needs to be? Mothers are supposed to love their children, care for their children, sacrifice for their children. But Mum hadn't done that. Cathy could argue that abuse had to look like bruises and broken bones, but she didn't have any idea what it felt like to have lies ingrained in your head.

The children were asleep as I shoved the double pushchair into the hallway. The room was spinning. Even when I sat on the stairs I was still falling.

Chapter Thirty-Seven

Narcissistic Rage

I laid Blossom in her cot, her legs so long that she almost reached the end. Only moments ago she was a baby, rocked to sleep in my arms, but at eighteen months she could settle herself. Bailey was lying on the floor in the lounge, his box of superhero figures spread around him.

'I've got to make a boring phone call,' I said. He turned from his game and looked up at me with his bright blue eyes. 'What are you going to do?'

'I'm playing *Avengers*,' he said with a broad grin. 'The Hulk is fighting Nick Furry.'

I suppressed a chuckle and nodded. 'Lovely. I'm in the kitchen if you want me.'

I'd been waiting all morning to make this call, trying my best to be present for the children, the unmentionable black cloud in the background since breakfast. It had been a short text from Mum, *just to say* that Sarah, the Parkinson's nurse, wanted to speak to me. I could imagine Mum was delighted that I'd been pulled into her medical affairs and I knew what was going to be said: I wasn't taking Mum's condition seriously enough. I felt exhausted at the very thought of someone else accusing me of failing my mother.

I sat down at the small table that we'd squeezed into the kitchen. We'd lost our dining room to the children, creating a brightly coloured, toy-packed playroom. I scanned my messages to find the right number and listened to the dial tone.

'Ah yes,' Sarah said, her voice firm and matter of fact. 'I saw your mother yesterday.'

I imagined Sarah was in her fifties, with highlighted hair and a long sharp nose: a nurse who'd seen it all, now sitting on a swivel chair at her desk with Mum's medical notes on the computer in front of her.

'We had an emergency meeting with your mum yesterday. She came with her friend – Sandy, is it?'

Mum had been telling me about this appointment for days, the growing excitement and anticipation of more medication, tests and doctors. She'd been most upset when Sandy refused to push her in a wheelchair to her appointment, though she'd walked unaided, nonetheless.

'Your mother has been presenting increasingly severe symptoms,' Sarah went on. 'Shaking, shuffling, weight loss. Have you noticed it too?'

'Yes, of course,' I said, making notes on the back of a bill. 'More recently though I've noticed she's becoming a bit… sort of, odd. Paranoid, you know? She imagines things. Her speech has become slurred.'

'What we realised when we observed her,' Sarah said, ploughing on, 'was the symptoms she is displaying are… Well, they're not real. What I think she may have done is googled a more severe version of Parkinson's Disease and imitated it. The shuffling, for example, it isn't consistent. And anyway, it isn't how people with Parkinson's shuffle. The same with her shaking hands.'

I dropped my pen. 'Yes!' I blurted. 'It's been happening for a long time. And her symptoms disappear as soon as she pops a pill in her mouth.'

Sarah tutted. 'Which isn't how it works at all.'

I couldn't catch my breath, a cool river of relief flooding down over me. 'I didn't think so. It's like she wants to be ill, and more ill. She loves seeing you. She loves getting more tablets.'

'Oh yes,' Sarah agreed, her exasperation clear. 'And unfortunately, we've been medicating based on the symptoms she's shown us. We don't expect people to exaggerate how unwell they are. And now she's suffering the ill-effects of having medication she doesn't need. As you said – the paranoia, the slurred speech.'

'Oh, I see,' I said, quickly scribbling some illegible notes and feeling a weight fall off my shoulders. I hadn't lost my mum after all; it was due to the medication. All those strange encounters were drug induced. 'Did you explain this to her yesterday?'

There was a hesitation and Sarah inhaled. I could hear her squeezing the truth into professional-sounding sentences.

'Both myself and my colleague met with your mother yesterday.'

I knew that Mum would've been thrilled to have them both there, especially in front of Sandy, the seriousness of her condition finally being recognised. I could imagine what a shock it must have been for her to realise that they were there to confront her.

'It seems she's been seeing one of us and then the other. Playing us off each other,' Sarah said through gritted teeth. 'We told her that we are taking her off almost all of the medication. Obviously, we'll reduce it slowly, but within a month she will be on the lowest dose. Back to where she started.'

'That's great news.' Though it was true, I doubted my voice portrayed it.

'Yes,' Sarah said, her tone echoing mine. 'But I'm afraid your mother didn't take it that way. Not at all, in fact. She shouted. There was a lot of bad language. Her friend tried to calm her down, tried to point out that this is good news. But she was insistent that we were to give her the prescription she wanted. I'm putting it down to the high levels of medication, but obviously this isn't behaviour that can continue.'

I could clearly imagine Mum giving a violent reaction, though I couldn't remember her throwing a tantrum before. It was as if I had cloaked knowledge that this was exactly what happened when

Mum didn't get her way. I bit my lip. Was I being told this as her appropriate adult? Was I supposed to feed this back to her like the parent of a rebellious teenager, and threaten the removal of her mobile if she couldn't speak nicely to those in authority?

'You can call me if you have any further concerns about your mother and, now that she's given me permission to share her medical information with you, I'll keep in touch.'

'Thank you,' I said. 'That's really helpful.' I felt my shoulders drop. Finally, someone in authority knew what was happening. It wasn't down to me to find Mum help now; the details were in her medical record and she was the responsibility of the nurse and the doctors. I could rest assured that all I had to do was feed them information of Mum's latest escapades and they would get her the help she needed. I gave a nervous laugh. 'I thought she was going mad, so it's reassuring to know it was the medication.'

'It's been an odd episode, but this should be the end of it,' Sarah said. 'Her initial diagnosis was correct – it's a mild version of Parkinson's – and she won't be affected by it for another ten years or so. Once she's on the proper level of tablets, then she'll be back to normal again.'

My mum was going to come back, that's what Sarah said. I wrote it down on the bill and underlined it several times. Normality would be resumed within a few weeks and it was all going to be okay. I'd realised that Mum was inclined to make out things were worse than they really were to get some more sympathy, and that was an understandable thing to do. It had worked while she'd had ME because it was such an uncertain illness with no tests or check-ups or ongoing treatment, but the Parkinson's had caught her out because it wasn't like ME. Having been confronted by the nurses, with Sandy and I as witnesses, Mum would realise she had to be totally honest in the future. It was perfect timing – she had the chance of a fresh start in the Lilly Fields, leaving the silliness of the past and her reliance on illness behind her. A whole life was waiting with new friends and activities and plenty of safety and help. She could visit the hairdresser's in the complex, go to the bar or the spa, enjoy day trips to the seaside and go to the restaurant any time she didn't feel like cooking. She could have a totally normal life.

Yet there was a nagging doubt, the sprouting seed that wouldn't die back, the question that remained: what did normal look like for Mum?

Chapter Thirty-Eight

The Flat

The receptionist at the Lilly Fields was so short that I couldn't see her over the desk until she stood up and smiled, her light pink lipstick matching her floral blouse.

'Oh dear,' she said, her voice trilling as she put on her thick spectacles and held a sticky note close to her nose. 'It says here your mother is too ill to meet you. But I can let you through the security door. Sign in there.'

Peter and I exchanged a knowing look and signed our names. This was how it was going to be then, from the very first time we visited Mum's new flat. The move had gone well, although Mum had done no further clearing out of the house. The contents of her semi-detached had been boxed up and squeezed into the two-bedroomed flat in the corner of the complex. She'd been quite perturbed that the movers had touched her underwear.

'I'm looking forward to seeing how they've got it all in,' Peter said. 'It's got to be a feat of engineering.'

We hadn't planned Christmas until a few weeks earlier. I'd dreaded talking to Mum about it, fearing the inevitable tears and tantrums. Only a bad daughter would make her widowed mother spend Christmas on her own, but neither Peter nor I could face another year with her after the disaster of the previous one. In the end it was Mum who'd brought Christmas up in conversation, ignoring my stumbling, nervous excuses.

'Oh good,' she'd said. 'That's what I was hoping you'd say.'

I'd felt immobilised, unable to swallow, my heart barely beating. It wasn't the response I'd expected.

'There's so much to do here,' she enthused. 'There's a whole party in the bar on Christmas Eve. And so many of my friends from the bank are here – Brian, do you remember him? Then there's Christmas dinner in the restaurant and that will be wonderful. And anyway, where would you all stay? You can't fit into my flat, there's not enough room. And if you think I'm going to cook for you all! I'm far too ill to do that.'

It was a surprise to me to feel so rejected. I didn't want to be with Mum on Christmas Day, but I hadn't anticipated that she might not to want to be with me. *It was good*, I'd told myself. She was starting to settle at the Lilly Fields, fully embrace the new start that it promised. *It was good.* So why didn't it feel good? There was a dark, harassing voice in my head, telling me she was playing a game.

We'd arranged to visit Mum the weekend before Christmas, so we arrived with a boot full of presents and all of us dressed in our nicest clothes – Blossom in a red velveteen Mrs Claus dress and Bailey in a smart polo shirt and jumper.

We walked towards Mum's flat, the hallway an imitation of a tree-lined street with intermittent flowerbeds. Down the centre of the passage ran a boules area which was fenced off with a low rope that Bailey stepped over without hesitation. Despite being enclosed it was as cold as the December air outside.

'Guess what colour Granny's new door is,' I said as we walked down the hallway.

'Greeeeen!'

'Or'nge!'

'Ah no, it's blue. Granny will be pleased. That's her favourite colour.'

We used the gold door knocker and waited in the long, dead street. If I'd known she'd take so long to reach us, I'd have kept my coat on.

'Do you think she's gone out?' Peter said, crossing his fingers behind his back and grinning.

'Has she, Mummy?'

'No, I'm sure she's in. Let's knock again.'

The door edged ominously open to reveal Mum, dressed in a freshly ironed red and black tartan midi skirt with a cream blouse, her hair newly styled. She grasped onto the door.

'Did you get my message at reception?'

'Yes. Hello, Mum.'

'I've been so excited for you coming,' she said, as the children scurried past her. 'But I've been so ill this morning. I couldn't even get out of bed.'

I stepped through the doorway, determined not to entertain her drama. 'This is lovely,' I said. 'It's much bigger than I expected.'

'Do you think so?' she said, gazing around. 'I think it's very dark. Very gloomy.'

'You could maybe use a lamp in here, but the lounge! Sunlight pouring in.'

'You should see it when it's cloudy. Dark, it is,' she said, following the children.

Mum's flat was small but perfectly designed, her neutral-coloured lounge as large as our own but stuffed with belongings. Already she'd lined the walls with furniture, onto which were piled an array of papers and records, books and photographs, ornaments and knick-knacks. Though we were given the tour of her bedroom and kitchen, the small second bedroom was entirely off limits, too full of boxes to step inside.

She gave the children some presents and lay back on the sofa, staring at the ceiling. Bailey and Blossom excitedly unwrapped clothes in the wrong size, playdoh that Mum vetoed in case it ruined her new carpet, and a large chocolate Santa that I whipped away to preserve lunch.

'Aren't you going to open any of your presents?' I said, indicating the large bag that sat by her side.

'Oh, well, no,' she said, wiping her brow. 'I didn't realise we were doing presents.'

I was trying to ignore how thin Mum was, in case I gave her any undue praise. Though she appeared to be wearing the same clothes as always, her arms and face gave away her weight loss. She was a bag of sharp bones sticking out of paper-thin skin but, rather than upsetting me, I was infuriated. I knew she was purposefully starving herself. She'd love it if I commented on her weight, but I wasn't going to be sucked in and acknowledge it out loud.

She stood up suddenly. 'Let's walk along the high street and go for lunch,' she said. 'I want to show you all off. Especially Blossom. Look at her in that beautiful dress. Gorgeous.'

'Bailey's smart too,' I said, turning to him as he beamed up at me.

'Oh yes,' she said, flicking me away. 'But Blossom – stunning!'

'Are you sure you're feeling up to it?' Peter asked, and I held my breath. 'I thought you were too ill to meet us at reception a minute ago?'

She strode towards the door. 'I'm better now,' she declared. 'That's what Parkinson's is like.'

I wasn't going to argue. For one day I didn't want to be the bad guy; I wanted to have a nice time together. We ambled down the street, Mum scanning the flats for occupants as we passed. Catching the eye of an elderly man a few doors down, she waved frantically and indicated he should open his front door. He kept it on the latch, clearly reluctant to entertain her.

'This is my family,' Mum said, inching towards the open crack.

The man nodded towards us. 'Hello,' he said. 'I'm afraid you can't come in. My wife is sleeping. She's not very well.'

'But they don't come very often,' Mum protested, pushing forwards.

I nudged the children to keep walking. 'Come on,' I said, as the door was quickly closed in Mum's face.

We walked down the self-styled high street with faux shop windows for the hairdresser's and convenience store. Four portly older ladies were seated on wooden benches as if they were overlooking the sea, gossiping on their holidays. Just out of the hairdresser's, they were smart in their A-line skirts and scoop-neck cardigans, the odd one out wearing wide-legged trousers and a long tunic. Though their wrinkles confirmed they were much older than Mum, they were dressed decades younger.

'Hello,' they cooed as the children passed. Mum whipped around us to stand proudly beside Bailey.

'Aren't they gorgeous. How old are they?' the lady in trousers asked Mum.

'Oh! They're… umm… one and two,' she stammered.

'She's a good walker for one. And he's so tall.'

'Blossom's almost two and Bailey's three and a half,' I interjected, smiling my best fake smile.

'Blossom was born on April Fool's day!' Mum said, and the ladies began to laugh.

'No, she was born in February,' I corrected. The ladies frowned at me in confusion, and I smiled even more sweetly though I was burning inside. Mum didn't falter.

We occupied a large table in the centre of the restaurant, the room decorated with tinsel hung from the ceiling. We pulled crackers and ate, Mum quiet and composed, conversation strained. It was a relief to see Sandy as we returned to reception. She was effortlessly chic in cream slacks and a baby-blue jumper, wrapping her arms around us in turn so we all smelt of Chanel no 5.

'Look how big you've grown,' Sandy said to Bailey, 'Such a smart young gentleman. And Blossom, what a lovely dress you're wearing.'

'Santa.' Blossom grinned, holding out her skirt.

I turned to Mum, but she'd walked on to the ladies who were sitting on the bench, away from Sandy.

'How's it been?' Sandy said to me in a low voice.

'She wouldn't meet us at reception,' I said. 'Was too ill apparently.' We both glanced at Mum as she gesticulated wildly. 'But apart from that it's been okay.'

'Listen to her,' Sandy said, shaking her head and turning her back on Mum. 'Can you hear her telling them she's got ME, Parkinson's and dystonia? You know what the nurse said about the Parkinson's and the dystonia, and as for the ME—'

'Talking about me, are you?' Mum said, scooting between us. 'What are you saying?'

I withered, my head dropping to inspect the floor as I scurried to find an excuse.

'I was saying you're telling those ladies about all your illnesses, Ellie, but I was there when you saw the nurse. She said you've got years until the Parkinson's affects you. And as for the dystonia, she said it wasn't real.'

My cheeks burned. I wished I could face Mum like Sandy without fearing what would happen. And what did I fear? What did I think she'd do?

Mum crossed her arms. 'She didn't see me at my worst,' she said. 'And you obviously haven't either.'

'It's like you want to be ill, Ellie,' Sandy said, mirroring Mum. 'And here, look, you've got a beautiful family you could be enjoying rather than thinking about those things.'

'I do enjoy them,' Mum said, grasping my arm. 'Anyway, it's no good, you'll need to take me back to the flat.'

I glanced over to Peter. 'I'll wait for you here,' he said with a knowing look.

I led Mum back down the high street, through the double doors and past the bowling green. She sat back in her armchair in her flat surrounded by presents and flowers.

'It was lovely to see you,' I said. 'I'll call you – what did we say? Half two on Christmas Day?'

'Yes, I think so,' she said, closing her eyes. 'Can you let yourself out?'

The children were rearranging some leaflets in reception when I arrived, Peter pulling a fake grin.

'How was it?' he asked.

I shrugged, ready to head home. 'It could've been worse.'

Chapter Thirty-Nine

The Game

I listened to the phone ring and ring. It was the sixth time I'd called, and I knew that the game was in full swing. I had known it from the first time I called – at half past two on Christmas Day – the dark, harassing voice telling me that I had walked straight into my mother's carefully planned trap.

It was Blossom's second Christmas, our first alone as a family, and up until then it had been perfect. We'd eaten what we wanted when we wanted, we'd opened our presents without rolled eyes or disapproval, we'd enjoyed Blossom and Bailey's excitement without the fear of a dramatic scene to turn the attention away from them. But all of it had been overshadowed by the last two hours of worry. I knew I was being played, but my imagination was doing somersaults as it drew up all the possibilities of self-harm Mum might have indulged in. I sat in the shadows of my bedroom, the dim December light already fading, and dialled Julia's number.

'I know she's causing another drama,' I said. 'But no one's answering at the Lilly Fields. Could you check on her? Sorry, I know it's Christmas Day.'

Downstairs again, I tried to concentrate on the new toys the children had unwrapped. Blossom was swirling in her *Frozen* costume while we built Bailey's marble run. But I wasn't really there; I was in the waiting room, knowing there wouldn't be good news.

'We've found her,' Julia said at half past five. Her voice was slow and calm down the phone. 'It's rather a long story. I couldn't get in the flat, but the manager let me in. Elinor was on the floor by her bed when I found her. But before you feel worried, darling, you need to know she had a pillow under her head and the TV remote next to her and she looked very cosy. She was warm all over, right down to her toes, so she hadn't been there for very long. She was dozy, like she'd drunk a bit too much alcohol, or maybe she'd taken something like Valium.'

Julia took a deep breath, as if the next sentence was hard to say. 'Look, Helen, it was a very controlled environment. The light was on, but her curtains were closed. She was saying she'd been there for two days, but she hadn't wet herself, she wasn't cold and she didn't have any pressure sores. In my nurse's opinion, she'd been there for three hours at most.'

Cloistered away in the darkness of my room, I pulled the duvet up around my shoulders as I shivered. From the moment Mum had said she didn't want to spend Christmas with us, I'd known she was preparing to throw another drama.

'We called the paramedics,' Julia said, 'and they've brought her into hospital. Sandy's here with me and Annette too. We all agree she's acting very strangely.

'When it's just us in the room, she's sitting up in bed, full of vigour – almost hyper I'd say. But as soon as the doctors walk into the room, she slumps down in bed, acting very ill, unable to move or speak properly. And then the moment they leave, she sits back up and is full of excitement.

'"You know," she said to us, "this is so wonderful. I'd much prefer to be in hospital than be at the Lilly Fields over Christmas."'

'She's starting to tell us that she hasn't eaten in a week, but I know she went out for dinner twice over the weekend, so that's not true.' Julia coughed. 'She wants a full-time carer.'

'Ah,' I said, slouching down. 'So that's where this has been leading.'

'Who are you speaking to, Julia?'

It was Mum's voice. Julia must have walked back to the side room while on the phone. I could hear the bleeping machines, the chatter of nurses, almost smell that clinical smell.

'Helen?' Mum was on the phone suddenly, as if she'd snatched it from Julia's hands. 'Oh, it's been awful!' she said with trilling excitement. 'Has Julia told you what happened? I was out cold for eight hours.'

'Yes, Mum,' I said. My voice was hollow, but I couldn't change it. She was purposefully ruining four people's Christmases and she was pleased about it. 'I knew this would happen,' I muttered, biting my lip, but she didn't hear me.

'It's been horrendous. I'm in agony. I've got carpet burns all over my knees.'

'Why have you got carpet burns?'

'From crawling on the floor.'

'I thought you were out cold?'

'I was! For two days!'

'You said eight hours?'

'I'm going to need a full-time carer now.'

'Why would you need a carer?'

'I don't know. It's probably my medication.'

'I'm going to contact your Parkinson's nurse. I think you need to see a psychiatrist.'

'I've got to go. The doctor's coming!'

I could imagine her dropping the phone into Julia's hands, falling back on her pillows, touching a weak hand to her forehead just in time for her medical review.

'This is what it's been like,' Julia confided. 'No consistency, no sense. They've tested her to the hilt and all they can find is a slight UTI. There's no clear cause for her to have been lying there for – well, however long. It keeps changing whenever you speak to her.' Julia's footsteps echoed down the corridor. 'I spoke to the matron and she says it's clearly all made up. They want her back in her flat as quickly as possible because the more help she has the less she'll be willing to do. I'm sorry, darling. This is awful for you. I don't know what she thinks she's doing.'

Somehow, even then, I knew where this road led. But she was my mother and I loved her, despite all of this, so what was I supposed to do? I had to follow her.

Elinor's Diary

1st January 2015
Last year I moved from my home of 42 years into a retirement complex. Helen had rung round to find me on Xmas day. I was in hospital from Christmas day PM. Julia found me. Dehydrated hungry ill not much was done to relieve this. No extra drinks. Only had 3/4 cheese sandwich on Christmas day. Christmas beyond me this year. Didn't do all my cards. Shopping was thanks to Annette as internet useless. On 23rd shaking all day long don't know why. Judy came and shocked. So asked her to help me clear up and get to bed early 5pm! The next thing was an ambulance man saying 'hello Elinor I've got Julia here' and I was gently woken to hospital. Had this from Helen after a traumatic New Year plus No Christmas due to UTI infection. The story is that I fell out of bed and was unconscious in my room. After an extensive search Julia and Ambulance found me. To hospital where I was given antibiotics. Worked hard to get walking back. Believe to have laid on my front with my left hand under my chest. Struggling to live. Not got much support and walking and doing anything V. hard. Will I recover? I don't know how. Tired. 'Carers' working but not much help really. Started year V badly when I collapsed. Turns out it was a bacteria UTI. Left me on zimmer struggling to live with people coming in 3 times a day to supervise. Confused.

Chapter Forty

Fresh Start

I thought I was going to have a mental breakdown. I didn't know what that looked like; all I knew was I couldn't take any more. It wasn't depression, it wasn't anxiety. It was the weight of balancing everything and getting nowhere. Running life at home with two children under four was hard enough, but the month of constant phone calls detailing my mother's latest dramatic escapades was unbearable and I thought I was going to break. Having carers had not fulfilled Mum's love of attention. It only seemed to have ramped up her desire to prove to everyone that she was 'desperately ill'. There had been daily emails, text messages and phone calls harassing me with Mum's latest crises, the illogical conversations, the bizarre symptoms.

Mum had called Sandy to ask for a meal to be brought round because she couldn't walk to the kitchen.

'Where are you?' Sandy had asked, as Mum's voice echoed around her flat.

'I'm in the kitchen,' Mum said.

Mum had told Annette that she needed help to go to the toilet but that the carers at the complex were ignoring her when she pulled the emergency cord.

She told Sandy that she'd had another fall and 'they' – the unnamed controllers – were telling her she needed more help.

She told Julia she kept 'freezing' – her phrase for standing like a statue, unable to move. Julia suspected Mum had been busy googling more symptoms to imitate.

It didn't seem to matter to Mum that it was all so obviously faked. She was being sucked down an inescapable vortex, the tales growing taller the less we believed her. Every day brought a new drama and I lived in constant fear of the next episode, the next round of crises I'd have to deal with. And what if I couldn't deal with it? Who would look after Mum if I didn't? She'd been discharged from the hospital, and though she was being visited by a spectrum of healthcare workers – an occupational therapist, the district nurse and a social worker – as well as paid carers who daily helped her get out of bed and take her medication correctly, this only seemed to pander to her desires. No one was dealing with the root cause of Mum's problems and nothing was said to explain what the root cause was. I was the only one trying to get her the help she really needed, and the same panic I'd felt at ten rose up in me: I was entirely responsible, with no one else to rely on.

I stood making lunch while the children imitated me using their toy kitchen in the playroom. It was the usual variety of toasted cheesy pitta bread, carrot-flavoured toddler crisps, grapes cut into halves, fromage frais and raisins. I longed for the day they'd eat sandwiches.

'I've made your lunch, Mummy,' Bailey announced, holding out a wooden frying pan with a plastic roast chicken and a kiwi fruit.

'Oh lovely, thank you,' I said, pretending to eat. 'Is there a drink too?'

'Tea, Mummy,' Blossom said, passing me a pink toy cup.

My phone rang from my pocket, the familiar buzz making my stomach drop. It rang too often now, the pings making my heart thump, my shoulders tighten, my hands shake. I could feel the next drama coming, my anxiety growing in preparation.

Annette's voice was grim. 'I'm sorry to be the bearer of bad news,' she said. I carried the plates of food to the table and lifted Blossom into her highchair, mobile balanced under my chin. 'I thought you should know. I'd arranged to go round to see your Mum yesterday afternoon.

But when I arrived, she was on the floor in the kitchen. She had a cushion under her and was leaning against the table. She'd knocked over her zimmer frame – I don't know where she's got that from.'

'Sounds set up,' I said, filling two cups with water in the kitchen. It was hard to generate real concern after the number of phone calls I'd had during the past month.

'I called a carer,' Annette continued, 'and we helped get her into bed. I told them it was possible she'd planned it as she knew I was coming. I said to your mum, "What happened?" and she said, "Well, I staged it." I was obviously a bit cross! I said, "Why did you do that?" and she said, "I don't know. It seemed like a good idea at the time." This isn't normal, Helen.'

'I know,' I said incredulously, scraping butter across a piece of toast for my own lunch. 'Sarah says she's sorting it out.'

'If she doesn't, then you must push her. You must be in touch with Sarah ASAP.'

I buzzed with frustration. Did Annette think I was sitting back and not doing anything? I'd contacted Mum's GP, I emailed Sarah every few days and I'd lobbied for a psychiatrist to be involved, but nothing was happening. What more could I do?

'After we'd got your Mum into bed, she said she was alright and wanted to go to the café. We got to the front door and she literally threw herself backwards. It was so obviously done on purpose! She hit her head on the door frame and we ended up having to go to A&E to have her injury glued. You know, love, she would have made an amazing actress. She was in the wrong profession.'

My futile laughter bounced around the walls, coming back to me even emptier.

'She's telling people she had a skull fracture, but I was there! She does use such emotive language to dramatise the situation. I don't know what can be next for her. I checked with the carer, and they never ignore emergency cords, so that whole thing about needing the toilet must be fiction too.'

I took a bite of toast. It was another lie to add to the list.

'It's not nice for any of us,' Annette said, though I didn't believe she really understood how bad it was for me. 'The other day I told her she would be better off spending her money on seeing a psychiatrist rather than on these carers. She hung up on me.'

Annette didn't realise that for Mum, putting the phone down on someone wasn't a casual impoliteness. Mum believed hanging up on someone was the worst possible offence. She may as well have used the F-word. It seemed that the magnitude of this statement had been lost on Annette, the finality of the choice Mum was giving her: she was to accept the behaviour or lose the friendship.

'Look, Helen,' she said. 'What she needs is to see you and the children.'

I put down my toast and watched the butter melt. 'I can't do that. Imagine if she purposefully injured herself like that in front of the kids.'

Annette puffed, as if I was being difficult. 'Then you need to go on your own if you're not willing to take them with you.'

I cleared my throat as if to cough away her tone. It wasn't about my willingness; it was about Mum's unpredictability. I wasn't going to risk my children.

'It's not that easy,' I said. 'I've got no one to have the kids.'

I didn't know why I was giving another excuse. Surely the first reason was enough.

'You need to arrange some childcare then,' she said, as if it were simple. 'If she sees you she'll be alright. It's a cry for help.'

Though I didn't believe that visiting would change anything, I didn't question that I was responsible for Mum's health and happiness. Neither the GP nor the nurse were intervening, so I needed to arrange professional help for her. I had to be the point of contact to string all the strange occurrences together and pass it on to the healthcare workers, though it didn't seem to get us anywhere. As much as I wished I could walk away, I had to look after her.

'How was she when you left her?' I asked, trying to change the subject.

'Oh, a different woman. Not even using the walker. Talking sense, sorting things out, all positive and laughing. I've told her I'll go round there tomorrow – see what we find then.'

It'd been almost a month since she'd gone into hospital and Mum had fitted a vast number of dramatic incidents into those thirty days. She was supposed to have got better when she moved to the Lilly Fields, but she was worse than ever. I didn't recognise her any more. For so much of my life, I'd believed Mum was intelligent and logical, confident and beautiful, kind and loving. I'd thought that everything about her was perfect and everything she'd done had been the best. It'd been driven into me so hard that my thoughts were taken captive. April was the best month to be born. Getting married at twenty-five was the correct time. Five foot eight inches was the ideal height. These weren't opinion; these were facts. I'd seen Mum as the thoroughbred horse, while I was the runt, staggering in her wake, trying to copy her despite my intrinsic faults and failures. But now, though a shadow of the mum I once thought I had still remained, my eyes had been opened – painfully wide – and Elinor was coming into focus for the first time. I'd been blinded, unable to see her for what she was, and now I couldn't forget what I'd seen in the light.

It was a relief when Sarah, the Parkinson's nurse, visited Mum at the end of January. That day I'd had a banging headache, so I'd taken pages from the newspaper and sticky taped them onto the kitchen floor for the children to colour. I sat on the floorboards while Bailey and Blossom giggled, unleashed to fulfil their dream of rebellious colouring, bright felt tip smeared up their arms and across their hands.

'Hello, it's me,' Mum said as I answered my mobile.

Amongst all the phone calls I received, these were the ones I dreaded the most. When Mum rang, the conversation often ended up with her shouting at me because I wasn't playing her game correctly. I should have gone running to her side on Christmas Day, but I hadn't, and still hadn't.

'Sarah came round on Tuesday. Just turned up on the doorstep, unannounced.'

I listened quietly, trying to assess her mood. Sarah wasn't drawn in by Mum's manipulations either. Turning up without an appointment was purposeful, to prevent Mum creating a crisis like she did whenever she was due a visitor.

'She said all the tests had come back clear.'

'That's good,' I said, tiptoeing gently.

'Yes,' she said.

There was no reason for her to have had a fall. No reason for her to have lain on the floor for – was it hours or days? The negative test results should have scared Mum. Not knowing why she had fallen should have upset her. But then again, Mum knew what had happened better than any of us.

'Sarah says she's going to continue to lower my meds,' Mum said. 'But it won't affect the Parkinson's unless I stop taking the tablets for a whole week. I couldn't believe that, but I suppose we'll see.'

'That's the same as your first diagnosis, isn't it?' I observed, stepping a bit heavier.

'Hmm,' she murmured, and I knew that idea was being dismissed. 'Sarah was very firm with me. Said I had to stop making up illnesses and faking falls and enjoy my life. Not that they were all faked, just that one. But anyway, it's been flagged on my notes that I'm not to be admitted to hospital for a fall.'

She said it so matter-of-factly, as if she didn't understand that she was being called a liar and a time waster, deaf to the implications.

'Sarah said I was a capable and able woman,' Mum said, her voice swelling with pride. 'She said that someone who can go out for lunch with her friends doesn't need carers. She said I can go out with my friends and do what I like. So, I've got permission now.'

'Lovely,' I said, knowing the sarcasm would be lost on her. I leant my head back onto the radiator, the warmth soothing on my shoulders. 'Are you going to get rid of the carers then?'

'One step at a time. I think I need them for about ten hours a week, to help me get going. But I've been for lunch with Annette this week and shopping with Sandy too and we had a real laugh. I bought a lovely new dress.'

'And no zimmer frame?'

'No zimmer frame. And how are you all?'

It had been a bad month, but there was light. The obsession with illness was coming to an end. Sarah had given Mum a good shake up and soon the carers would be gone. A corner had been turned, Sandy said. I've got my friend back, Annette told me. My mum would return to me. I would go back to being a normal mummy, not torn between two generations. And, in time, I would visit, and Mum and I could have normal mother-daughter time together.

Elinor's Diary

7th January 2015
My friends and family gave me talking to telling me to be truthful about my PD. Shocked hurt – alone.

Chapter Forty-One

The Last Time

My footsteps echoed down the Lilly Fields high street, rhythmically tapping out *Bailey, Blossom, Bailey, Blossom*. The children were home with Peter while I visited Mum, trying to look forward to spending the afternoon together, trying not to dread it. I'd done my best to anticipate any criticism – my hair up as she liked it, simple jeans and a baggy jumper to deflect any comments about my weight.

We'd arranged to meet at reception. But when I arrived, she didn't answer her mobile. She didn't come walking down the promenade, standing tall, without her stick or the walking frame. She hadn't left a message at the front desk. It was ominous silence. Though I'd hoped for better, I'd known deep down that this would happen. I should have turned around and gone home that minute, but instead I stepped up my pace when I saw someone going through the security doors and walked down the cold, tree-lined street, my heels the only noise in the empty corridor. Mum's blue door was ajar, and I crept into the flat, the hallway steeped in darkness.

'Mum?'

'Helen? Oh, Helen. Thank god you're here!'

She was in the lounge, the long strip of light that slipped through the half-drawn curtains cutting the room in half. Draped across the floral sofa, she'd gathered peach cushions to prop herself up, a glass of water and a drained coffee cup on the table beside her. I noticed she'd done her make-up and her hair was perfectly permed into ashy curls.

'I'm desperately ill.'

'What's happened?' I asked, standing in the doorway, my legs unwilling to take me any further.

'I've been working like a black.'

The words were a smack to my face, a punch in my stomach. This wasn't the normal language she used, nor the type of phrase I heard amongst my family or friends. It was jagged, disgusting, appalling – not just because it was unacceptable racism. I didn't recognise the person saying it.

'Mum!' I shot. 'You can't say that.'

'Well, I have!' she wailed, raising her hands. 'I haven't had anything to eat or drink all day.'

No, I thought, *not this again.* Everyone had said she was better. We were going to have a nice mother-daughter lunch together and go shopping and be normal. There weren't supposed to be any more lies, any more drama.

'You'd better go to bed then,' I said. 'I'll come back another day.'

I wouldn't have begrudged leaving, even after the two-and-a-half-hour drive. I'd rather have gone home to Peter, Bailey and Blossom, back to a life that made sense.

'You've got to help me,' she said, her blue eyes pleading with me. I forced my legs forward, perching on the sofa beside her, my hands clawed together.

'Come on,' I said. 'Let's get you to bed.'

She raised a limp arm. 'I can't,' she protested. 'You'll have to carry me.'

'I can't carry you,' I scoffed, standing up again. 'Why don't you take my arm and I'll guide you.'

She shuffled around, sitting up with both feet planted on the floor. 'In a minute,' she said, as if this action had taken all her energy. I sat back down on the sofa, tracing each pained expression on her face.

I'll leave soon, I told myself. *I'll get her to bed and then I'll go.*

She lay her hands onto her lap. 'It's no good,' she said. 'I can't get to bed on my own.'

'Yes you can,' I said, using the same voice I used with the children to get them to put their shoes on. 'Remember what Sarah said. You are a capable and able woman. You don't need a frame or carers. You can do this.'

'I can't,' she said. 'You have to help me.'

'Is this a new dress?' I asked. It was the same distraction technique I used when Bailey got frustrated. She sat up a little and gave a strained smile, her hands curled around the smooth, wooden arm rest.

'Yes, I got it with Sandy,' she said, admiring the black and white polka dots.

'Lovely,' I said. 'Did you have lunch with her too?'

'Yes. At the Castle… roast dinner. I had prawns for starters and trifle.'

'Prawns and trifle? That doesn't sound good.'

She raised another weak smile which slowly transformed into a grimace as she shuffled towards the edge of the sofa.

'No one understands how ill I am. I'm so desperately ill. No one cares.'

'We all care,' I said. 'Me and Sandy and Julia and Annette. We're so glad your Parkinson's is only mild.'

It was inch by inch, but I could see her creeping forwards as if she was going to stand up any moment. Soon I could leave.

'And there's the ME.'

'You said you don't have ME any more.'

'No, I don't.'

She was right on the edge of the sofa, balancing precariously, her feet on tippy-toes ready to take her weight. I stood up ready for her to follow my lead.

'Come on then, let's get you to bed.'

As if in slow motion, she dropped herself down to the floor, gripping the arm rest so she moved as steadily as possible. A controlled move, it brought her gently onto her knees before me.

'Did you see that?' she said, with a large, watery blink. 'I fell off the sofa.'

I stifled a laugh. 'No. You lowered yourself onto the floor.'

'No, I fell.'

This was comic, wasn't it? One of those hilarious real-life moments. But it didn't feel funny. It felt perverse.

'Mum, stop it.' I took her arm lightly to lift her up. 'Let's get you to bed.'

Her scream ran through me and I stumbled backwards towards the door. She was wild, her teeth like a jackal's, her tongue sharp as she spoke. She was possessed now, her face altered.

'I see,' she spat, pointing a finger at me. 'I'll have to crawl on my hands and knees, will I?' She held me with her piercing eyes, detailing my reaction as she dragged herself towards me. 'Look at what you've done to me,' she said. 'You're trying to destroy me.'

I was fastened to the floor, mute and open mouthed, my pulse pounding. She was coming towards me, each movement exaggerated and purposeful, a tiger prowling towards me. Then her face sank, and she cried dry tears, her mouth wide and wailing. No longer predatory, she had instantly changed to pathetic.

'Oh god!' she said to the ceiling, 'Take me home!'

I stuttered, fumbling backwards. 'What would Sandy say if she saw this? I think we should call her and tell her... tell her what you're doing.'

I fumbled in my coat pocket, my sweaty hands sliding my mobile from my grip. I pounded the keys, unable to pick the correct options. Everything was blurred.

'Sandy, I'm at Mum's. Please talk to her. She's crawling across the floor. She says she's desperately ill...'

'Ooh, what's she doing now?' Sandy asked.

I held the phone up to Mum who snatched it from me and grasped it to her ear. That fierce jeer returned, fastening on me while she crouched, ready to pounce. If anyone could talk her down it was Sandy, her best friend for nearly thirty years. She'd listen to Sandy, listen to her calm, confident manner, listen to the logic she was undoubtedly speaking.

Mum's high-pitched scream was as unexpected as the first time. It threw me backwards into the doorway.

'You're cruel!' she shouted.

She threw the phone to my feet and I grabbed it automatically, feeling the bile rise in my throat as I bent down. I needed to get out.

'Right, that's enough,' I said, trying to sound stronger than I felt. 'Stop this ridiculousness right now.'

She didn't speak, glowering at me intently, the tiniest curl at the corners of her mouth. She knew better than anyone that I was incapable of walking away from her. Each grasp of the carpet, each dragged leg movement, was made slower and larger.

'You little bitch,' she seethed. 'Look what you're making me do.'

I dialled Peter next and gave Mum the phone again.

'Ooh, you!' Mum hissed into the mobile. 'You horrible man! You've never believed me.'

I took back the phone.

'Get out,' Peter said. 'She's fine. You know she's fine.'

'She's hysterical. I don't know what to do.' I dropped my voice to a whisper and stepped into the hall. 'I'm scared, Peter, she's scaring me. What do I do?'

'Leave. Walk out and leave her.'

'I can't!' I sobbed. 'I can't. She's my mum!'

'You can. I give you permission. Leave.'

I didn't leave. I couldn't leave.

'I'm going to make tea,' I said to Mum.

I closed the kitchen door behind me, leaning on the wall and trying to calm myself down. I took long, deep breaths but my hands were trembling, the sweat dribbling down my collar. There was no one else to call, no one who could help me. The noise of the kettle had drowned out Mum's wailing, but it was coming to the boil too quickly and I didn't know what to do. I made the tea as painfully slowly as I could and waited until there was quiet. Cracking the door open I could see Mum on her hands and knees in her bedroom, opposite. She stood up and got into bed like she usually did, as if nothing had happened.

I closed the door carefully and took another deep, unsteady breath. I needed to get out. I picked up the same patterned teacup we used to drink out of while we watched *Watercolour Challenge* after school and carried it carefully into the bedroom. I was seven again, carrying the first cup of tea I'd ever made. I drilled my eyes onto the lip of the china to make sure I didn't spill it, but the cup was too heavy and my hands too shaky.

Mum was back to normal. Her face wasn't sharp or accusing, her mouth back to its thin pink line. She was sitting in bed, cushions propped up behind her, the pale duck egg covers neatly folded around her waist.

'Oh, tea, lovely.'

I stood away from her, close to the door, while she gulped down the drink.

'What time is it?'

'Twelve.'

'Is that all? What shall we do now then?'

My mouth was desert dry. 'I thought you were "desperately ill",' I choked. 'Needed me to carry you to bed. You crawled across the floor…'

In an instant it was back again, that terrifying glare, that changed face. 'I'm your mother,' she said, each word laboured. 'I've done everything for you. I paid the nursery fees.'

I stared at her, my eyes too wide. I knew what she was saying, I knew it was a threat. I had to take her insane histrionics because she had bought me and my children. She owned me. And it was true – she had paid for the children's nursery, but it was something she could easily afford and wanted to do. And then she'd stopped the payments without warning, as if she were punishing me.

This was a new game – money as manipulation – one I didn't have the rule book for. I ran through my memories, searching for something to link this to. My parents had paid for my university fees and my wedding, but they'd said it was their pleasure, something they'd saved for over many years. They hadn't held it over me, a debt to be repaid in the future. They were gifts.

Now I thought about it, though Dad was generous with his finances, Mum's attitude had been different. She loved to boast about the price of things she'd bought and made a note of how much others spent on her, including me when I was a child. Her favourite hobby was shopping, and she bought racks of new clothes – though they were all dowdy, outdated styles. But she also saved up the cooking fat in a tin pot that lived in the fridge, made her own yogurt in the airing cupboard and hoarded broken belongings in case they were useful one day. It was a mixture of rabid middle-class consumerism and post-war make-do-and-mend that had kept me on my toes in my childhood; were we financially secure or not?

She put down her teacup. 'Oh,' she said, her attention abruptly deflected to her hands. Her eyes darted around the room. 'Where's my wedding ring? Oh! Where is it?'

She was instantly morphed into a victim again: soft and vulnerable, in need of a rescuer. Her shoulders were slumped, her eyes filled with worry and she was back in the persona of a frightened, old woman. I picked up the gold band from her bedside table.

'Is this it?' I said. She grabbed it from me, holding it up and kissing it repeatedly.

'My darling Alan. I love you, I love you!'

It was too exaggerated to be real, a superstitious act, a dramatic imitation of what she thought someone who loved would do. It made me think that she didn't love him at all. It wasn't the first time the thought had crossed my mind. I remembered how she had moaned continuously about caring for Dad as his health deteriorated, as if he were an inconvenience. When he lay dying in hospital, she had been reluctant to visit him, keeping away for weeks because of a sore throat. And, despite her dramatic collapse when he died, I couldn't remember seeing her cry, not on that day or any other. The pieces didn't form a picture of a devoted, loving wife.

'Did you see that?' she said, turning to me again. 'I loved your father. Really loved him.'

I pinched my lips. It was a poor forgery of love, an ugly, disturbing display. Mum hadn't noticed me pull away from her. She replaced the ring on her finger and drew back the bed covers nonchalantly.

'It's too early to go to bed,' she complained. 'Let's go for lunch.'

The room was dark, though the curtains were open and the day still light. I needed to leave.

'I don't know who you are,' I said, backing out of the room as if pulled by an invisible string.

'Where are you going?' she said, sitting up straighter. 'You're supposed to be here to spend the day with me.'

'You need to rest,' I muttered. I swiped my fingers across the hallway wall just to feel something solid. 'I've got to go home.'

I could hear her calling me as I shut the front door, but I didn't stop walking once I was out of the flat. My calves ached with my swift steps as I bolted down the corridor and, on the high street, I broke into a run. I ran, though I hated running, my footsteps beating on the floor as I passed reception, not stopping to sign out or make small talk with the lady on the desk. I burst outside and the fresh air shocked me, the cold sting of exiting a night club drunk. I groped for my keys, pressing the button to unlock the car before I reached it, my head throbbing, my chest heaving. Mum might have gone out of her back door; she might have beaten me to my car; she could be anywhere.

I fell into my Fiesta and locked the doors. There was a stitch in my side. My chest was icy with shallow, ripping breaths as if I'd torn my lungs apart. I didn't want to look around in case she was near, but I didn't want to stay. Too faint to drive, I sat with my head in my hands, overtaken by dry sobs that rocked my whole body.

I was afraid, I was afraid, I was so afraid.

I was never going back.

Chapter Forty-Two

Microwave

'Why are you calling me?'

I was a dog going back to its vomit, trying to make something out of the mess that was left. It had taken me three days to work up the courage to ring Mum, waiting for a moment when Bailey was in pre-school and Blossom was napping so I could speak to her alone. I had expected apologies or at least excuses.

'I was wondering how you were after the other day.'

I'd practised saying this sentence to make it sound fluent and neutral, but I knew my quavering voice gave me away. If I hadn't realised before, it was clear to me then that I'd always been afraid of her.

'Well… well, I don't know.'

I'd caught her off guard. I didn't know what she'd expected, but this wasn't it.

'I'm very ill,' she said. 'I've slept solidly. But I need a new microwave, so I'm going to get one later. And Christina from the bank is coming to help me sort my paperwork.'

'I hope you feel better and have a good day.'

'Yes, well. We'll see.'

Neither of us realised, but we'd set the tone for all our future conversations. Neither of us was capable of doing anything more than dither around the edges of the truth. I wished I could pour out my anger, my confusion, my annoyance that I was having to pay more attention to her than my own little children. But she was my mother, so I had to keep taking the phone calls, updating

Sarah, nagging the GP and crying in the kitchen, while she played her games.

It was almost Blossom's second birthday, the cloud low as we trudged home from Bailey's pre-school. We'd settled into the new routine – the school run in the morning, the walk home for lunch, the children's afternoon nap. Bailey was wrapped in a mossy-green parka, my arms around him as he stood on the buggy board, both our gloved hands clinging on to the pushchair. Blossom refused to wear gloves because it stopped her sucking her thumb, the cow-print blanket pulled up around her.

'I think it might snow,' I said, noticing the stillness of the day.

Bailey looked up at me. 'Can we build a snowman?'

Pushing the two children up the hill took all my strength, and beneath my enormous coat I was drenched in sweat. At home the heating was raging, and Blossom began to cry because she was too hot. Bailey was already de-robing, shedding layers that were scattered across the floor. I quickly stripped Blossom down to her leggings and a jumper. She toddled away leaving me amongst the mountain of discarded clothing.

'Mummy, when's lunch?'

I pulled off my shoes and abandoned them at the front door. My phone rang as I hung my coat over the banister, a number that I didn't recognise. 'Hold on,' I called to the children.

'Hello, Helen,' said the nervous and unfamiliar voice. 'You don't know me, but my name's Christina. I used to work with your mum in the bank.'

I went into the kitchen and opened the fridge, the cool air blasting me as I noted the lunch options.

'I'm sorry, I know this is a bit odd,' she said with a nervous laugh. 'I got your number from your mother. I went over there today, and a terribly strange thing happened. I thought you needed to know.'

I'd never met Christina, but I pictured her as a short lady with permed hair and glasses. She sounded sweet – the sort of person

Mum could easily manipulate. I went into the lounge, turned on the TV for the children and went back into the kitchen.

'I went to her flat today, as we'd arranged, and the door was open,' Christina said. I was tight-lipped, knowing that this small detail indicated the sport had begun. 'Elinor was calling for help from her bed, saying she couldn't walk and needed to be helped to the toilet. And I was shocked. I've known your mum since she was a sprightly young thing in the bank and to see her reduced to that, old before her time, unable to care for herself. I mean, she's younger than I am. I helped her shuffle to the toilet. I practically carried her. Helped her to do her business. What else could I do?'

'Oh no,' I said, waiting for Christina's embarrassment to rise into condemnation that I, her only child, had not been the one there, helping Mum urinate. I was ready with my excuses, ready to tell her that it wasn't what it seemed.

'She told me,' Christina continued, 'that she hadn't had a hot meal in days. Said she couldn't cook anything for herself because her microwave is broken and she's unable to get out to buy a new one. I said, "It's no trouble, no trouble at all." I'd pop out to town, get a new one – it wouldn't take half an hour. As it went, the roads were clear and the shops were deserted, so it was even quicker. Only twenty minutes and I was back.' She gave a little chuckle that I reflected back to her as I cut up some grapes to stay the children's hunger.

'But when I got back, the door to the flat was wide open. I was really worried, because I'd taken the key so I could let myself back in and I thought, *Who could have opened the door?*

I could picture it all so clearly, Christina approaching the door, cautiously entering the darkness of the foyer, uncertain what she'd find.

'And there was your mum, standing in the hallway. She didn't realise I was there to start with because she was talking to a young man who was fitting a new phone line. She was standing there chatting away to him, virtually dancing around him, making jokes and *flirting*. A completely different woman to the one I'd taken to the toilet twenty minutes earlier. You can imagine how I felt. Absolutely mortified. I couldn't get out of there quick enough.'

I watched the children from the doorway as they mechanically put one grape into their mouth without moving their eyes from the screen.

'It's not right,' Christina said. 'I don't understand.'

'None of it's right,' I agreed, moving back into the kitchen for the inevitably long conversation. I hoped it wouldn't snow so I couldn't disappoint the children again.

There was limited solace in knowing that even Mum's acquaintances could see right through the lies. The bombardment was crushing me. I was imitating normality, flitting from a world where life involved taking Bailey to pre-school and playing with Blossom to a life where nothing made sense, and no one would help me. My requests for Mum to see a psychiatrist had been translated into a handful of phone calls from the NHS counselling services, who'd quickly decided Mum was lonely and could be discharged. I was desperate. No one was taking in the bigger picture. No one was listening to me, and I was running out of options to garner help. I didn't know who to call or who would even take my calls. I was alone, sinking, unable to find someone who knew what to do.

I was busy packing the nappy bag the next day, ready to go to the garden centre with Blossom for a free morning out, when I got an email from Julia. Mum had left her an answerphone message: 'Julia. You might like to know that I have had several falls and I'm now in hospital. Could you phone my solicitor please? Oh actually, I suppose I could phone him myself.'

As I read her email, another one pinged into my inbox. Sandy had received a strange phone call minutes earlier.

'I'm in hospital!'

'Are you?' Sandy said. 'How are you calling me from your landline then?'

The phone went dead. Caller ID must be a bitch when you're trying to lie. I read the emails as I sat crouched on the floor beside my bag. What did Mum think she was doing? Had she really lost all sense of truth and logic? My mobile rang.

'Helen, I'm not well, not well at all,' Mum said.

'What's happened now?'

'The GP has been out to see me because I have a severe chest infection.'

I inhaled deeply. It was cruel. Dad had died from emphysema and I knew the sound of someone struggling for breath. I knew that sound to his death bed.

'You don't even sound wheezy.'

'You would say that,' she scoffed. I imagined her crossing her arms like a sulky child, pouting her lips at my refusal to join in. 'You must be very dissatisfied with your whole life.'

'Why's that then?' I said, rising up with my temper.

'You think I've lied about being ill. You've turned against me.'

'Oh, and you've never lied about being ill, have you?' The tip of the volcano was brimming in my voice.

'Never!'

'Not when you faked that fall and told Annette you'd made it up.'

She paused, but only for a moment. 'That was once.'

'Ah!' I said, standing straighter. 'But then how can I believe you? If you've done it once, you're willing to do it again. And as for the whole scene with Christina—'

'How do you know about that?' she said, as if it would be impossible for Christina to dare tell on her, though she'd asked Mum for my number.

'She rang me!' I stormed. 'I get strangers calling me because of your erratic behaviour. You know you can't see Bailey and Blossom while you're like this, don't you? Especially after the way you behaved last time I came over.'

'What do you mean?'

'When you were crawling across the floor, shouting obscenities, slamming the phone down on Sandy. And then ten minutes later you wanted to go out for lunch.'

'I don't know what you're talking about,' she said.

I was bubbling over, unable to withhold my frustration any longer. She couldn't really believe that we were all falling for her manipulations, could she?

'You've forgotten, have you? That's convenient.'

'Ooh you little…! That's unkind, that is.'

'Because I've caught you out?' I exhaled noisily. 'You know I love you, Mum, and I don't want you to be like this. You need to see a psychiatrist. And until you sort yourself out, you can't see the children.'

I'd been waiting to tell her this, trying to find the right moment to say it without upsetting her. This wasn't what I planned – throwing it at her in an argument, trying to threaten her into getting real help.

'You're banning me from them, are you?' she said. I could hear her outrage that for the first time ever I was putting boundaries on what I was willing to give her, a limit to what she could have from me.

'What would you do in my position?' I said, lowering my voice. 'If your mother had crawled across the carpet and shouted swear words at you, would you have taken me round to see her when I was a child?'

'No, of course I wouldn't,' she said, and I blurted out a laugh. She was an intelligent woman, but so tangled in lies that she'd caught herself up between wanting to tell me what a good mother she was and trying to convince me she was a stable person.

'There we are then.'

I could hear her writhing in her own web. 'But that's not fair! I don't remember that happening.'

'You don't seem to remember lots of the appalling things you've done. Doesn't mean they didn't happen.'

'It's this terrible disease, Helen. It's the medication, the hallucinations.'

It was a run of excuses, a dodging of responsibility, a classic move of turning pathetic when cornered. I'd not only read about these narcissistic traits, I'd lived in their wake for thirty years.

'That's rubbish,' I said, with uncharacteristic confidence. 'I know what Sarah said. She said you have mild Parkinson's. That you could be off your meds for a week before you notice side effects.'

She took a deep breath. I wished I could have felt pleased that I'd won the argument, but I felt as knocked down as ever. Having cornered her, I feared what would happen next. I worried that having been caught out by her lies and exaggerations she would run away. She might decide to disappear and start again, find a whole new group of people to manipulate. She could tell them that everyone had deserted her and she was all alone – play her favourite role as the victim. And I'd never know where she was or what she was doing, if she was safe or if she needed me, and it would eat me alive.

'I don't know what to say to that,' Mum said, having found her tactic. 'That's astonishing. Sarah has never said anything like that to me.'

'Stop it!' I said, banging my hand on the wall in another eruption. 'You say you don't pretend to be ill but in the last half an hour you have called Julia, Sandy and me with three different made-up crises. You told Julia and Sandy you were in hospital. Did the GP even visit?'

I needed her to see sense, to come out of this cloud of nonsense. But you can't bottom a liar.

'I can't talk to you when you're like this,' she said. 'You're tying me up in knots, trying to catch me out. I don't know if you've noticed but I am not well. I've got to go to bed. Goodbye.'

Elinor's Diary

16th February 2015
The ME group said I was talked down to – like a little child.
Had words with Helen. She says she doesn't want me to have
anything to do with the children till I've seen a pycologist. So
mad at 4pm rang for taxi going to spend spend spend. But
Annette phoned me and reminded me of pill so she drove me
to M&S and I bought 5 pairs of pants to throw away 5 old
pairs. Horrible text messages from Julia accusing me of all
sorts of things. Discovered lots of work to do addressing people.

Chapter Forty-Three

Brainwashing

Bailey had decided he would be going as Captain America to Jake's fourth birthday party. His costume, complete with pumped-up muscles and a mask, hung by his bed. Blossom was struggling to decide if she wanted to go as Spiderman or Supergirl. It was a tough decision because she wanted to be like Bailey, but the sparkles on Supergirl's tulle skirt were beguiling. She stroked the dress sombrely as my phone rang. A few years before I would have looked forward to speaking to Mum. How quickly things had changed.

'I've been totally cleared,' she announced. 'I've seen the shrink and passed the test with flying colours.'

'Oh,' I said, my chest tightening. I didn't even know she had an appointment. Had it been on the phone like the NHS counselling services – a brief conversation where Mum could twist the circumstances and play the eternal victim? Or, if it had been face to face, maybe she was lying about his findings, which would hardly be a first. Unless the psychiatrist had missed it. My hands were shaking. After everything that had happened – the inconsistencies, the illogical conversations, the terrifying dramas – how could he have missed it? She must have gone alone, kept the appointment quiet from her friends as well as from me, and made sure she was in control of the story. She must have played the naive, middle-class, disabled widow and manipulated her way out of the truth. However it had happened, she'd been found sane, and I'd lost my excuse to keep the children away from her.

'You can reduce the carers now,' I said, playing my final card.

'I like having carers,' she said. 'Although I know better than they do. They tried to give me my meds early yesterday and *I had to tell them* when they were due.'

I gave a nervous chuckle. 'If you know better, then you should cancel them. Why can't you take your own meds?'

There was a long lull. I helped Blossom out of her clothes and into the Spiderman costume. She pulled the mask down over her wispy blonde ringlets and raised her hands in fists.

'It's all Carys's fault.'

'Carys? What's this got to do with Carys?'

'The whole reason I have carers is because of Carys,' Mum said. I could picture her striding confidently through her house, assured that she was speaking the absolute truth. 'She gave me the wrong number of tablets at the pharmacy and I took them, and now they're saying I'm incapable of taking my meds correctly and need carers.'

'Who's "they"?' I said, furious that she would lie and endanger Carys's job at the pharmacy. Didn't she care about anyone but herself?

'Sarah.'

'Sarah told you to *cancel* the carers,' I said as firmly as I dared. 'She said you're an able and capable woman who should be enjoying your life rather than focusing on your *mild* condition.'

It had become my mantra.

'It's a degenerative disease, I've got to keep on top of it. I saw Sarah today anyway,' she said and sniggered. 'She found out I've had all sorts of professionals from the hospital visiting me since I was discharged in January. It's been lovely. But she's cancelled all that. She found your dad's medical notes on my bed too. Said I shouldn't have them and took them away.'

Studying Dad's medical notes and gathering as much professional attention as she could was a far more believable story than the last. I helped Blossom undo the Spiderman costume and pull on Supergirl.

'Anyway, I can come and visit now. That's what you said.'

I fastened Supergirl's cape and walked decisively to the kitchen, mustering a stern voice. 'No, I'm sorry, you can't. You're too erratic. And if you're ill enough to need carers five times a day, then you can't take a holiday.'

I listened to her huff, her victorious mood dampened. 'Didn't Annette talk to you? She'll come with me and be my carer.'

Annette had continued to encourage me to visit Mum, preferably with the children, even after the crawling episode. I didn't know how she could justify the situation to herself or how Mum could manipulate people into seeing things from her twisted perspective. She'd repeatedly treated Annette badly, used her and lied to her without the slightest attempt to disguise it, and yet it felt like Annette still viewed me as the problem. It was infuriating sorcery. Mum had conjured me into the stubborn villain, cruelly refusing to see her desperately ill mother, when the truth was that I was unwilling to compromise the safety of my family. I wished Annette could see through Mum's lies.

'You need to get on an even keel,' I said as Blossom flew around the kitchen, her cape blowing out behind her. 'I can't have you coming here and talking to Bailey and Blossom about how many falls you've had, like last time we called you. You didn't even ask how they were.'

'And I don't know what Christina was talking about.'

She had become deaf to me, a different conversation running in her head. Or was it part of her clever control, the moulding and manoeuvring of the situation to make my head spin?

'She said I was unpredictable,' Mum continued. 'But that's what Parkinson's is like. You're bad one minute and completely fine the next.'

I wished it was late enough in the day to have a glass of wine. 'That isn't what it's like, Mum. We've been through this over and over.'

'That's the other thing I wanted to ask you,' she said. I sat down heavily at the dining table and put my head in my hands.

'I overheard my carers yesterday. They were standing outside my kitchen window. They'd put me to bed, but obviously I'd got up when they'd gone. It was only eight, after all. They were saying, "I don't know why we're coming. She's getting all this help and she doesn't need it. She's brainwashing people. It's all made up."'

I lifted my head but said nothing, my heart pumping fiercely. Bailey was chasing Blossom with a shield he'd made out of sticky tape and a cardboard box, both of them laughing raucously.

'I thought it was interesting,' Mum said into the void. 'You know, a totally new idea. I wondered what you thought about that.'

Was this a trick? She sounded calm, curious if anything, as if she was asking me my layman's opinion on some scientific theory. But she could turn; I knew that too well. Should I agree with the carers and risk pushing her away? Or continue my useless, gentle tactics?

'Well… you know… that's what we've all been saying to you… me, Sandy, Julia. You're not ill.'

'I'm not in contact with Sandy and Julia any more.'

'That doesn't surprise me. Not after the way you've treated them: shouting abusive language down the phone at them, all those made-up falls.'

'What do you mean?'

'You know what I mean. We've talked about this a million times.'

'I don't know what you're talking about.'

'You do. Making a scene when people arrange to visit you. Throwing yourself backwards. Hanging up on your friends. Pretending to fall. Pulling the red emergency cord.'

'This is a big shock.'

'Mum, stop it,' I said, my cheeks burning. 'What about the day when I visited, and you crawled across the carpet.'

'I have no knowledge of that,' she said, as if I'd reached an answerphone.

'Yes you do,' I insisted, opening the back door, brushing Bailey and Blossom outside and away from me. I didn't want to shout at them for making happy noises, I wanted to shout at my insane mother; but I wouldn't do that. 'You crawled across the floor saying all sorts of horrible things.'

'It must have been a mental breakdown. But I'm fine now.'

It was a politician's prepared answer: a quick response to an accusation she knew was coming and couldn't get out of without claiming insanity.

'The fact that you say you can't remember any of this means you're not fine, doesn't it?' I said, hoping that the possibility of another line of illness, another means of getting medical attention, might at least appeal to her.

'This is a very big shock,' she said, robotically. 'I'm going to have to lie down.'

In the garden, the children were running circles around each other and laughing as the phone went dead. If this was Mum's version of sanity, then how had the psychiatrist missed it?

Elinor's Diary

30th March 2015
Psychiatrist came here. Very informative. Turns out the only person in danger from me was ME! Went to buy slippers. Hotter lady escorted me to Taxi Rank as I looked so pale. Good time. Went to lunch with Annette. Ate Ostrich – stopped pill working!!! Don't eat game.

31st March
Sarah came and assessed me – think I'll be here for LIFE. Can't see a way out. On the other hand where will I go? Bad day shaking all day. Need more help.

8th April
*Rang Annette and asked if she wanted to take me to Jewellers
to have my rings cut off. Only 1 out of 3 would do it. Hurt
quite a lot and hard to do. Helen wasn't impressed when I
told her but at least we are talking. Later found she'd talked
to Julia and complained about me UNFAIR. Strange that
my friends cept Annette and a few others are telling Helen
all sorts of rubbish. Even Sandy is distant.*

Chapter Forty-Four

Gaslighting

Most days the soft play centre was rammed, the bright equipment filled with little legs and arms, shouts of delight and devastated tears, a mixture of childish voices, mummy chat and local radio. But on a Friday morning it was deserted, the usual clammy heat replaced with ice-cold air and the smell of stale sweat.

At the Friday toddler group, Cathy had continued to urge me to visit Mum with the children despite my protestations. Her apparent belief that mothers are always good was a brick wall between us. I felt she was ignoring my fears and concerns because she couldn't believe that a middle-class mother could be a bad parent, let alone an actively harmful influence and that it was my responsibility to look after Mum, no matter what.

I was in a hall of mirrors, and it was impossible to uncover who was telling the truth. I rocked from knowing that Mum was lying about her symptoms to thinking that Cathy was right and I was being a bad daughter. And if that was true, then Julia, Sandy, Judy and Annette must have been lying to me about what was really happening, trying to spoil my relationship with my mother for some unknown reason. Maybe Mum had been right and there was a worldwide united front wanting to bring her down.

I had to remind myself of everything that had happened: recall Sarah's conclusion that Mum's symptoms weren't real. I replayed all the strange incidents and remembered that I'd experienced them myself, while Cathy had not.

I'd read several survivors of narcissistic parents describe their childhood as being trapped in a dark cellar lit only by a flashlight, but I was drawn to Plato's cave to explain my experience. In his allegory, Plato imagined a group of people chained from birth in a cave, facing a blank wall. Behind them burned a fire, the only source of light, and all the prisoners could see – their only experiences of the world – were the shadows of a puppet performance put on behind them by their captors.

Mum had been my fire and my puppet master: the one controlling what I saw and how I saw it. Everything was portrayed through her perspective; some of the events were clear, made large and highlighted, while others were indistinct and blurred, mere contours beyond my reach.

The events since my miscarriage had broken my chains and I was finally able to turn around to see the show behind me. At first it had been impossible to believe, and I kept turning back to the familiar cave wall, hoping that I could ignore the new reality, unwilling to believe I'd misinterpreted my life so entirely. But once I'd glimpse the truth, it was impossible to ignore. I had no choice but to escape the cave.

I staggered into the blinding light of the sun – life outside of my mother's shadow play – blinking and confused by the new world I saw around me. Often I was unable to make sense of it, but I was beginning to realise that the normality of the cave I'd grown up in wasn't normal at all. The cave had never been a place of safety but a familiar prison. Still, I wasn't sure how to move on since my captor was my mum. It was impossible to escape her.

It was a relief when the Friday toddler group folded and I no longer saw Cathy regularly. Instead, every Friday after I dropped Bailey at pre-school, Blossom and I met Jemma and Lucy at a Soft Play Centre, walking through the doors as soon as they opened.

'Morning,' said the manager, her glum face backlit by a rainbow jungle mural behind her, happy pop hits blurting from the loudspeaker. 'One admission, one cappuccino and a jug of red squash?'

I gathered the shoes and coat Blossom had abandoned on the floor, wiping my face subtly and raising a weak smile. 'You know me so well,' I said.

Lucy and Jemma's girls were already on the slides, Lucy's youngest throwing rice cakes onto the floor from the highchair.

'You got the squash again,' Lucy said, as she unloaded her pushchair. 'I'll get it next time. Watch the baby while I get a coffee? You having a cob?'

'I'm thinking of a full breakfast,' Jemma said.

Lucy put a hand to her chest in mock surprise. 'Now there's a suggestion.'

'I will if you will.'

'I need to lose weight.'

'Bread's worse than protein. Helen, what do you think?'

I shoved a tissue into my pocket hastily and nodded. 'Let's do it.'

Lucy turned towards the counter, but Jemma examined me. 'Something's different.'

I smiled and brushed my hair behind my ears. 'Alright, eagle eyes.'

'Did you get your ears pierced?'

'I totally did.'

The tiny gold stars were shining badges of honourable rebellion. Mum had told me relentlessly that we didn't get our ears pierced. She hadn't, her mother hadn't and I wasn't allowed to. It would ruin our ears. We didn't want to ruin our ears. We didn't like earrings. Except I really did like earrings and had spent years gazing hopelessly in shops knowing I had no chance of owning them myself – even when I'd moved away from Mum and had my own job and my own life. I'd only decided a couple of days earlier that I was going to do it – a spontaneous act of defiance. I didn't want to be like Mum any more.

'They're so pretty,' Lucy said. 'Where did you get them done?'

'The place where every thirty-two-year-old goes to get their ears pierced.'

'A tattooist?'

'No, Claire's Accessories.'

Jemma's laughter filled the empty play centre. 'That's such a "Helen" thing to do. You need to get the biggest, brashest, sparkliest pair and wave them in your mum's face,' she said.

Lucy and Jem headed to the counter, and I sat with the baby munching beside me. I hated these moments when I was alone, my thoughts immediately taken to Mum. For four years I'd cried over Mum daily, a secret grief that I tried my best to keep hidden. Maybe I managed to portray being okay so well that Cathy thought the situation couldn't possibly be as bad as I was describing.

I had my back to my friends, so I let my tears fall, breaking holes in the froth of my coffee like raindrops falling into deep snow. Though I'd decided not to see Mum again, I'd continued to try to persuade her doctors to reassess her, desperately hoping for a breakthrough. I'd spent hours on the phone, sent tens of emails, but I wasn't making any progress. I'd run out of hope that Mum might get better or that I could do anything more. There was an impenetrable fortress built around her medical affairs: the NHS policy to protect the patient. In practice that meant that my opinion and my insights were repeatedly ignored. The GP might have taken my phone calls, but the psychiatrist wouldn't. His receptionist refused to let me speak to him and my emails disappeared into the ether. As the psychiatrist had signed her off, and Mum had the money to waste on carers for years to come, there was really nothing more I could fight for, even though Mum was getting worse.

That morning she'd called me as I was loading the dishwasher to tell me that she'd had her wedding rings cut off, although I already knew. During the previous week Mum had been telling her friends that her fingers were swollen – though it was clearly untrue – and had wrapped her rings with cotton wool to make them tighter. Annette had told me that Mum had bound her hands into fists for no apparent reason, and though Mum assured Annette that she'd been told to do it at A&E, Annette was certain this was another fantasy. Mum was now unable to unfold her fingers and had made Annette take her to the jewellers for the rings to be removed. Funny how Mum had no shame to tell me that she'd destroyed her most precious link to my dad, while I was too afraid to tell her I'd had my ears pierced.

'Have you thought any more about the power of attorney?' she asked.

'I've already told you, Mum. If you want it, you have to arrange it. I went to my solicitor like you asked and they said I can't do it. It looks like I'm forcing you into it. You need to talk to your solicitor.'

'Oh right, another thing I have to do.'

'You're the one who wants it, Mum,' I said, shaking my head as I stacked multicoloured plastic plates. 'I don't see why you need it. Sarah said you could be living completely independently – you don't even need to be at the Lilly Fields.'

She huffed. 'I have a degenerative disease, Helen. In fact, I have three chronic illnesses.'

'That's not what the nurses say,' I said in a patronising sing-song voice. I didn't bother concealing my frustration any more since the conversations went round in illogical circles no matter what I did. I drained the milk from a breakfast bowl and stacked it in the machine before grabbing the next one from the counter.

'I've been fooling you, haven't I?' she said.

I was frozen, holding the bowl in mid-air. 'What do you mean?'

'I've been lying to you. To all of you.'

I put the bowl back down on the side delicately, as if making a noise might frighten away the moment of clarity. 'Lying about what? About being ill? So, you don't really need the carers?'

The interval felt lengthy, my ears straining to hear any indication of her thoughts, but there was only stony silence.

'Having carers attacks my weakness.'

Her voice was sucked dry of drama with neither her usual endgame whine nor giddy pleasure at her own manipulations. I couldn't decode what sort of game it was.

'What weakness? Do you mean the carers give you attention for being ill?' I said, the words plodding from my tongue.

'And having the cord here. I pull it and they come running.'

'So, none of it has been true?'

'I need help, Helen.'

I could barely breathe, tortured relief choking me. I could have collapsed with tears, screamed with excitement, but I didn't want to scare her back into the madness of the previous years.

'You need a psychiatrist,' I said, amazed at how calm my voice sounded. 'This is so good that you're admitting it. You need to call your GP and ask them for help. And then we can go back to normal.'

'Okay,' Mum said, and I could hear her genuine smile. 'I'll do that now. Thanks, darling.'

It was the best conversation we'd had in many months. She'd called me darling! I punched the air as we said goodbye and danced around the room, the children joining in curiously. And then I finished the dishwasher, dressed the children, took Bailey to school and waited. The GP might move quickly; the psychiatrist might get her the real help she needed; normality might be around the corner. It wouldn't be easy, but it might be possible.

Mum called me an hour later as we were walking from school to soft play, Blossom quiet in the pushchair. The day seemed so much brighter than it had done earlier. My chest was thumping as I answered.

'So, what did they say?' I asked.

'Who?'

'The doctor.'

'The doctor?' she said with derision.

My stomach dropped, my voice falling low and slow automatically. 'Yes. You said you were going to call the doctor.'

'Why would I do that?'

The low cloud was hunkering down, making the air thicker and harder to breathe. 'When we spoke an hour ago, you said you'd been fooling us, lying to us. That you didn't really need the carers. That you needed real help. And I said you should call the GP, see a psychiatrist.'

In the pause my legs became weak. I wished I could sit down.

'I didn't say that.'

Did she know she was lying? Or was she so trapped in the lies that she'd completely lost her grip on reality? Did I speak to the real Elinor that morning, the one imprisoned in an inescapable cycle of attention seeking? Or was the real Elinor speaking to me now? I needed to talk to the unreachable psychiatrist.

'You did,' I said. 'We only spoke an hour ago.'

'No, I wouldn't have said that,' she said, strong and certain.

'You don't think you need help from a psychiatrist?'

'No, of course not.'

'But… but even though Sarah has told you that you are a capable and able woman, who has mild Parkinson's that won't affect your life for at least ten years… and yet you have carers! And even they tell you that you don't need them. You don't think that's strange?'

'Helen,' she said, and I could imagine her hard face: that assertive gaslighting look that forced me to back down. 'As I said, you need to understand that Parkinson's is a debilitating illness that will only get worse. Wanting carers is perfectly normal.'

'You're not going to contact the GP or cancel your carers?' I said, stumbling down the road towards the soft play.

'No, I need the carers.'

'They're not "attacking your weakness", like you said?'

She breathed out heavily, frustrated with me. 'In my right mind, I absolutely deny I ever said that. I am desperately ill. I need carers.'

I was sinking into the ground as she grew more defiant. My grief was ever present, covered lightly in tissue paper smiles that broke at the smallest touch, but this had torn through my ability to conceal it. Tears rushed down my face.

'Who are you?' I sobbed. 'I don't know who you are any more.'

Did she purposefully ignore my words and my tears? Or did she no longer hear me?

'There's someone at the door; I've got to go,' she said, cool and unrepentant.

Mothers always love their children, they always care for them, they always do their best. Mothers are always good.

'Oh, Helen! Are you alright?' Jemma cried, and I jumped. I'd forgotten I was in the soft play centre. She wrapped her arms around me, and I sobbed into her cardigan. I was being consumed, robbed of my own life and drawn into a world of labyrinthine darkness that my mother controlled – one which was destroying me.

Extract from Dr Brian Coldfield's Assessment of Mrs Elinor Page.

April 2015

Mrs Page is a 68-year-old lady with a lifelong tendency towards anxiety which has now worsened due to her Parkinson's Disease and in addition the Parkinson's Disease itself is obviously implicated in when and how she expresses her anxiety symptoms. Mrs Page's situation is one where the physical and psychiatric cannot be easily unravelled and I am certain it is best not to try.

Chapter Forty-Five

Care Home

The summer that Bailey turned four was blazing hot. In the photographs I took, the children were stripped down to their pants and coated thickly in sunscreen, jumping on the bouncy castle we'd rented for Bailey's party, while the adults sought shade. I snapped Blossom painting the fence with water and took some others of our new kitten, a mad tortoiseshell ball of fur which spun around the garden, chasing her tail. I pasted the photos into weekly emails to my mother, smudging my make-up as I pressed send. There was no response, though Annette told me Mum replied to other people's emails. Mum didn't answer my phone calls or return my messages either.

Less consuming than the previous months of endless communications from friends and acquaintances, Mum's lack of contact was a foreboding background buzz in my daily life. I didn't know where or how she was or, more worryingly, what she was doing. And though she was erasing me from her life, I was being held accountable for hers. The Lilly Fields called to say they couldn't cope with Elinor any more. She was having over a hundred falls a month and was often found by the carers, standing beside the red emergency cord and pulling it though nothing was wrong. They told me she would have to leave the retirement complex, but since I had no power of attorney or any contact with her, there was little I could do. And then, at the end of the final summer before Bailey started school, Annette emailed me to say that Mum had been taken to hospital after a fall. I was back to balancing phone calls to doctors while looking after my family.

The children were drawing with chalk on the patio. Bailey was using his new-found skills to carefully spell his name, while Blossom made as long a line down the paving slabs as she could.

'Look,' I said to the nurse in Mum's local hospital. I knew how I sounded, nothing like my usual persona. 'This is my fifth phone call. I need to speak to the consultant about my mother.'

'I'm sorry he's not available at the moment, but I can put you through to the matron.'

Matron's smooth south Wales accent was balm to my frustration. Finally I was speaking to a medical professional, other than Sarah, who would listen to me without making me feel like I was wasting her time.

'I'm sorry but he's not available right now,' she said, 'but I do understand what you're saying. The problem is your mother is refusing to get out of bed. She says she can't walk any more, which leaves us in an impossible situation. It's clear to all of us here that what you've told me is right, but the doctors have deemed she has mental capacity so we've got to do what she wants. We've agreed she'll go to respite care.'

I pictured matron sitting at a desk in a side office – a mature nurse who had probably worked in the hospital all her life. She had no airs about her, just sympathy for our equally cornered positions. 'She'll go into a county hospital, a sort of a care home, until she's back on her feet again. We've found nothing wrong with her so she should be back in her flat in no time.'

I would have liked to believe matron, but I knew that it was wishful thinking.

'I really don't want her to go to respite care,' I said. 'She won't come out again.'

'I agree,' matron said, 'but it's what she wants. There's nothing we can do.'

I knew that this signalled the end. Once Mum was in a care home there was no coming back. She would only spiral downwards.

I'd been too afraid to talk to my extended family about what was happening until then. I was scared they'd misunderstand me, dismiss my concerns as typical old age or give me that confused look that made me feel like I was being a bad daughter. I was afraid I was betraying Mum. It was only once she was in the care home and I was sure that I wasn't misunderstanding the situation that I dared call them.

I started with the relative I most liked, though we had little contact. My Great Uncle Reg was jovial but straight talking and had known Mum since she was a child. I told him not just what had happened in the last week and previous few years, but also what I'd discovered about the ME.

'Of course she's made it all up!' Uncle Reg said, laughing from deep in his tar-lined lungs. 'It was so obvious. When I saw the video of you all in America, with your Mum dancing around. All those places you went, all that walking! How could she have done it, with her disability?' He took a deep breath. 'I knew then. But it runs in the family, you know dear, this obsession with being ill.'

Next was Aunt Anita in her bungalow in the West Country. 'I'd tell your Mum to be positive, But all she wanted to do was talk about her illness.' She gave a little, thoughtful sigh. 'It went on for so long, I started to wonder.'

'You know, I've always suspected,' said Aunt Gwen with contrasting confidence. A petite lady with pure white curls, she had a rolling accent and a flat that smelled of Welsh cakes. 'She's been like this since she was a teenager. Every cold was the flu, every minor thing was a major illness. I used to worry about you. What your mum's disability would do to you.'

It was better than accusations, but it was depressing to hear that many of my relatives had known, or were pretending to have known, that Mum had been lying for all those years. It didn't reassure me to learn that they'd worried about me, since they'd chosen not to intervene in our isolated lives. I felt pummelled by their comments, the obviousness of Mum's deception a stinging damnation of my naivety.

I was being assaulted daily by flashbacks, memories rearranging in my mind. Happy Christmas Eves spent with Judy and Paul were stained with my mother's self-obsessed rants. The day the washing machine blew up wasn't a funny anecdote but a picture of a neglectful and uncaring parent. My belief in my 'good' childhood had become a distasteful mockery. It was so obvious when you knew. It was so humiliating.

I remembered my primary school project to design a new chocolate bar. Mine was called 'The Miracle Bar' because it cured ME. In secondary school I chose to use my public speaking homework assignment to raise awareness of ME, the ignored illness, and how the afflicted suffered. I didn't need to research my topic as I knew it all by heart. Mum must have been so proud that I'd swallowed her lies even when the inconsistencies were staring me in the face. She didn't even need to be subtle with me because I naturally trusted my mother. I was so desperately gullible.

'Did your dad know?' my rakish cousin, Robin, asked. Tall and dark with a thick beard, he had been the mysterious bohemian of the family. He mirrored my own unanswerable questions. 'How didn't we notice? And why would she do it? I mean, she's got so much to live for. She could be enjoying her grandchildren.'

There was only one person left to contact who didn't know the full story. I didn't have her number, but I didn't fancy another phone call anyway. Even if she didn't believe me, I knew I had to try to tell Judy what I'd discovered. It had been a year since I'd spoken to her last, when she'd told me to 'back off' my mother. So much had happened in the interim.

'Thank you for your letter,' Judy said. Her voice was soft, almost a whisper.

It was eight o'clock in the evening, a moment chosen carefully to guarantee my attention. I leaned over the back of the sofa and looked out onto the empty street, my hands shaking. *Worst case scenario*, I kept telling myself, *it will be one difficult phone call.* I'd had so many difficult phone calls, one more didn't matter.

'You know, I knew something wasn't right.'

Until then, I hadn't realised how tense I'd been. I was kidding myself about one difficult phone call. I knew the after-effects would have shamed me for days.

'I couldn't work out what was going on.'

Judy took a deep breath in, her voice uneasy. 'Last week I went to the nursing home and there she was, sitting in a corner in the lounge. Well, it's quite a nice little set up, TV and sofas, but all these old people. And there's your mum looking... normal. We chatted like usual – she told me how ill she was, how terrible the Parkinson's was – that's always the topic now. But I noticed the more sympathy I gave her, the worse she became. She started shaking and slumping down further in the seat – and this is over quarter of an hour or so. But the nurses completely ignored her. It didn't seem right. And then she told me you weren't visiting,' she said. 'Alarm bells were ringing in my head. Anyway, she managed to walk back to her room using the zimmer frame, and I left her there in bed. But I couldn't help thinking it wasn't right. I didn't know what to do. And then your letter came. All the pieces fitted into place. She's making it all up.'

Justification felt deeply satisfying – a glass of ice-cold cola on a burning-hot day.

'It's hard to believe, isn't it?' I said.

Judy had known my mother for forty years and for all that time the friend she thought she knew was lying to her, playing her, humiliating her. It felt like burning heat in your chest, like foundations being destroyed.

'I'm thinking back to when I called you before,' Judy said. 'When your mum told me how awful you'd been to her.'

'Yep, that was pretty bad,' I said, giving a stunted laugh. 'She was playing us against each other.'

'I can't believe it,' she said, her voice quivering. 'How did you feel towards me?'

'I was pretty hurt,' I said, deciding an enormous understatement was better than furthering Judy's embarrassment.

'I'm so sorry,' she said. 'I didn't know.'

'I knew it wasn't really your fault,' I said, standing up and going to the kitchen. 'She's very clever.'

'So manipulative. And a fantastic actress. Gosh, I'm absolutely furious with her! She's made a fool of me. You know, I really believed her.'

'We all did. We're all her fools,' I said as I poured myself a large glass of chilled white wine. There was a moment of quiet, but it wasn't awkward; rather a stunned silence.

'What do you think will happen now?' Judy's voice was quiet and thoughtful. 'Will she go back to the Lilly Fields?'

'I doubt it,' I said, taking a large gulp. 'She'll be thrilled to have full-time care. But I don't think she realises that in a nursing home she'll lose all her independence, all her control. Up until now she's been the one manipulating the situation. But with every move she makes to prove how ill she is, she limits her options to create drama.'

'You think she'll be there forever?' Judy said. 'At sixty-eight years old?'

I knew that sounded bad: an otherwise able woman choosing to live her remaining years in a care home. But I also knew that it wasn't enough for Mum.

'I think,' I said, rubbing my face, 'she only has one choice left to her if she wants to get more attention.'

I knew exactly what she would do next. I knew because it was second nature to her, an ability she prided herself on, a manipulative talent she'd used throughout her life to gain attention. I knew she would starve herself.

Chapter Forty-Six

A Normal Christmas

Life was very different by the winter of that year. In my normal, understandable world there had been momentous change. My little longed-for baby, Bailey, had headed out into the big world, our days now framed by the school run. In my other world, the side where the sun never reached, my mother had, unsurprisingly, not moved out of respite care. She'd spent three months in a care home, dramatically declining without any hope of intervention.

'It's such a waste of money,' Peter said, rolling up his blue work-shirt sleeves. 'Your poor Dad worked so hard to save, and she's frittering it away.'

'It's not that surprising,' I said, getting up from the table. 'She's destroyed everything else he gave her. And at least I'm not responsible for her any more. I know she's safe.'

'Did you speak to Sarah?' he said as he piled up the plates after dinner.

'Yeah.' I brushed some crumbs from the table into my hands. 'I said Mum'd gone from living completely independently to being bed bound, incontinent, losing weight rapidly and having these horribly bent joints in only eighteen months. Sarah said it wasn't that quick a change; people can go downhill that fast.'

'Yeah, sure,' said Peter. 'When they're actually ill.'

'Exactly,' I said. 'Apparently the GP visited again and didn't raise any concerns. But Sarah said she was very concerned,' I said, leaning against the door. 'She insisted the psychiatrist, Dr Coldfield, visit Mum again. And by the sound of it, he freaked.'

Peter shook his head and watched the washing-up bowl fill. 'I should think so. He was the one who signed her off and said she was no harm to herself.'

'That must seem pretty different now,' I said. 'He's referred her to the neurologist, and they've said there's a possibility it could be a very rare form of Parkinson's.' I felt my throat tighten. 'Maybe she's not absorbing her diet, which would explain why she's malnourished, but the home are saying she's eating fine. It could be something like a brain tumour. But it might be entirely psychological. They've decided it needs further investigation so she's going to Birmingham for tests.'

'No way,' Peter said, turning to face me. 'After all this time, they're actually going to do something.'

I nodded. 'She'll be seen by a specialist Parkinson's neurologist and a rehab consultant. Sarah says she's asked them to keep in touch with me.'

'Are you alright?' he said, pulling me into his chest.

'What if I was wrong?' I said, molten tears brimming. 'Maybe she hasn't been making it all up. Maybe she's got a brain tumour and her personality has changed. She needed my help and I've left her to rot.'

'But it might not be,' he said into my ear. 'It might be psychological. And anyway, how could you have known? You've done everything you could.'

When I was a teenager, there was a ride at the fair that Carys used to love. A circular room, it spun faster and faster until you became stuck to the wall, at which point the floor would drop away, leaving you revolving in mid-air. I felt like I was back there again, dizzy and groundless, uncertain what was true.

I'd heard stories of people whose personalities changed, their illogical choices destroying their relationships and lives, all caused by an undiagnosed brain tumour. It wouldn't be impossible for this to have happened to Mum. And yet, if that were true, then what about the ME? The last four years didn't seem like new behaviour, but an acceleration of what had already been. It was more like her mask had fallen off. But I was still plagued by doubts; maybe Mum had been right and 'they' were out to get her, and I was being played in a different game altogether.

I woke up each morning in the cold sweat of shame, but I didn't visit Mum. I doubted myself, but I didn't visit. I couldn't make sense of what was happening, but I didn't visit.

The tree had been up in the lounge for three weeks, the sparkling lights enthralling the children and tempting the cat to tug at the baubles. Peter and I had decided that, once the children were in bed, our new Christmas Eve tradition would be to wrap the presents while listening to Christmas songs and drinking a bottle of mulled wine. Before that could commence, I was cooking a ham. I'd never liked ham, but Mum made one at Christmas so I was mechanically following suit. An unknown number was calling me.

'Can I confirm you are the daughter of Elinor Page?'

I held my mobile under my chin as I covered the ham in cherry Coke, the apron Mum had bought me one Christmas, long before we had children, tied around my waist.

'Sorry, who is this?'

'I'm from the adult safeguarding team in Birmingham.'

If I were working at four o'clock in the afternoon on Christmas Eve in a stuffy hospital office, then perhaps I might have used staccato words and an aggressive tone too. But I was just a mummy trying to assemble a normal Christmas for my family.

'I'm investigating an allegation of abuse that Mrs Page has made.'

I clenched my jaw. Despite Sarah's assurances, this was the first time anyone from the hospital in Birmingham had contacted me. I'd endlessly called the number Sarah had given, but the phones were rarely answered, and when I did occasionally get through, I was told that I couldn't have the consultant's phone number because I was not the patient. Messages I left for him were never responded to, and all I could get were apologies that they couldn't talk to me because my mother hadn't given permission and she wasn't well enough to give her permission. She was, however, still capable of making allegations, something she was hardly unfamiliar with, and a sure sign to me that she was in control.

'Right,' I said. Christmas appeared to be her favourite season to throw her biggest stunts. It was very clever, very well planned. A typical narcissist's tactic. 'And what's the allegation?'

'Mrs Page has alleged that she was kicked at the care home where she was prior to being admitted to hospital. Do you know anything about this?'

I didn't even bother to hide my contempt. I reeled it off: a well-worn statement I was bored of repeating. 'My mother has a history of lying, faking falls and making allegations, so I very much doubt this is true.'

'Right.'

There was a long gap that told me he had not expected me to say that. It was supposed to have been a two-minute phone call to tidy up some loose ends before his Christmas break.

'When was the last time you saw your mother?'

It felt like a cruel, unnecessary question, as if he were judging how good a daughter I was, making me justify my comments on the woman I'd known intimately for thirty years. I heard a stinging accusation that if I'd backed away from my mum, then I couldn't really love her, couldn't really know her.

'Sorry? How is that relevant?'

'It's one of the questions I need to ask.'

I ground my teeth. 'A year ago.'

'I see,' he said, and I could hear he considered me no use to him. 'And you don't know anything about her being kicked?'

'No.'

'I'll be making further investigations.'

'And will I hear back from you?' I asked, already knowing the answer.

'If I need to speak to you again, I'll get in touch.'

I wanted to scream down the phone at him, tell him how hard I'd tried to get Mum help, tell him how many times I'd been ignored or told that this was my fault while, all the time, my life was being shaken like a snow globe into an unrecognisable flurry. But his lack of knowledge and insensitivity were the least of it. All these miles away and my mother was still managing to ruin Christmas.

Chapter Forty-Seven

A Full Physical Assessment

Mum.

It's so small: more of a sound than a word, the first hum on infant lips. I wished it felt that instinctive to use, but it was a fiery insult every time I tried to form it. I didn't have a mum, only a mother. Being a mum meant something more than the person who had given birth to me.

I hadn't given up on her though. I'd memorized the hospital extension numbers during the three months Elinor had been in hospital and spent hours with my mobile pressed to my ear while I did up buttons on coats, practised spellings, made packed lunches. Still, the only person who would speak to me was Sarah, the Parkinson's nurse, because my mother had given permission for her to share her medical details with me many months earlier. If it hadn't been for her, I wouldn't have had a clue what was happening in Birmingham.

'They've tested her for everything,' Sarah said. I sat at the dining table cutting out snowflakes ready for the third birthday party while Blossom, dressed in full Elsa costume and white-blonde plaited wig, re-watched *Frozen* in preparation.

'They fed her through a naso-gastric tube to correct her malnutrition and her weight returned to within the normal range. Tests showed no evidence of a disorder affecting the absorption of nutrients. But now she's off the feeding tube she's losing weight again.'

I continued cutting. Despite Sarah's authoritative voice, I knew from her lack of comment that this inconsistency wasn't passing her by. I wasn't sure how my mother was doing it, but she was starving herself under the noses of these doctors, the same ones who said they didn't think she was capable of making decisions.

'She's been given injections to loosen the contractures in her arms and hands, but they haven't made any difference, which suggests Mrs Page is deliberately holding herself that way.'

I traced the edges of the snowflake with my fingers. I wanted to reminisce with Sarah about the time my mother shouted in the office because she threatened to take away her medication. How simple it seemed back then. Now it was far beyond me, like a balloon that had floated from my reach, leaving me helplessly stranded, resigned to watching it rise away.

'The consultant, Dr Froome, reported that he has regular reasonable talks with your mother,' Sarah continued, 'but that whenever he tries to assess her memory she becomes deliberately vague and confused. He told me he'd asked her who the prime minister was, and she grinned at him and said, "Oh, I don't know, is it Harold Wilson?"'

I shook my head. 'She clearly knows she's lying to him then. She's not even hiding that she's pretending to be mad.'

'Quite,' Sarah said. 'The physical tests are the same. Mrs Page's reactions are inconsistent each time, suggesting she is fabricating her symptoms. She's been taken off all the Parkinson's medication and it hasn't made any difference, again suggesting she is, at the very least, exaggerating.'

I put down the scissors. I would have felt so ashamed of myself if my mother had been diagnosed with a brain tumour, but it would have meant that I could put the last few years down to something solid and logical. She'd spent months in hospital being tested extensively and the conclusion was that not even the Parkinson's was real. I didn't understand why, when faced with these results that showed she was lying, Elinor continued to fake it. Didn't she feel humiliated? She'd lost her friends, her family, even the support of the doctors and nurses whose attention she so desired. Pretending to be ill wasn't achieving what it once had, but she kept on, nevertheless. It was beyond logic, an addiction so powerful it was impossible to detach.

'There's one last test,' Sarah said. 'A specialist in rare presentations of Parkinson's is going to visit. He'll give Mrs Page a one-off "super" medication and, if she doesn't respond to that, it will finalise the verdict on her Parkinson's Disease diagnosis. Beyond that, the only treatment will be physiotherapy.'

'And what are the possibilities for my mother faking the results of the super medication?' I said, listening to Sarah give a chuckle.

'She can't influence the results. It's a yes or no, not something subjective.'

I carried on cutting out the next spiked, icy shape. 'Has Dr Froome got my messages?'

'Yes,' Sarah said. I felt the shutters coming down on the conversation. 'Psychiatric intervention isn't on the cards.'

'And the allegations of abuse?'

'I don't know what happened with that. No one's mentioned anything more about it,' she said, her voice chirpier. *Just a little fun for my mother then*, I thought, *to while away her second Christmas in hospital.*

We ended our call as I finished the snowflakes, and I quickly typed an email to Annette with the results, hoping they spoke as loudly to her as they did to me. I hoped she would see through Mum's lies but I didn't receive a reply.

My phone calls to the hospital had become infrequent once I knew what was happening. But since the doctors in Birmingham had decided Elinor was incapable of making good decisions about her health, they were only too pleased to call me repeatedly to get my permission to go ahead with treatment. For a fortnight I was in high demand, although most often from doctors who seemed to consider me a means to an end, not worthy of having my questions answered or my concerns heard.

I'd left Blossom to finish a jigsaw in the lounge when a hand surgeon called me. I wondered whether it would be Blossom, surrounded by puzzle pieces, or the doctor who would finish first. Blossom was, after all, a whizz at jigsaws.

'Could you tell me when the contractures in your mother's hands started?' he said, in a calm, well-mannered voice. In a few days he would be operating to prevent Elinor's nails from growing into her palms. I wondered if she was happy with what she'd done to herself.

'Yes, it was when she bound them up,' I said. I was making lunch, folding a piece of bread over the ham and cheese and listening to Blossom clicking the pieces into place. It must have been several seconds before I realised the doctor was speechless. I'd forgotten that Mum's behaviour wasn't run of the mill.

'Sorry, she did what?'

I winced. 'This is the fifth time I've told a doctor this,' I said. 'Isn't it on her medical record?'

'No.'

I sighed. 'She bound them up for no reason and they've seized up that way. It really ought to be on her notes. I've asked Dr Froome to call me so I can give him some history. I've asked many, many times. Maybe you could ask him again.'

'I'll pop it on Mrs Page's notes,' he said. Blossom took my hand and led me to the lounge. The finished picture was perfect.

'After this surgery, what's going to happen?' I said, giving Blossom a hug.

'We'll check her hand is healing and then she'll be discharged back to her local hospital,' he said, grasping onto something more normal.

'And that will be the end of her treatment?' I said, wandering back into the kitchen as Blossom began a new puzzle.

'From what I can see on her notes, yes. But I'm not her consultant, just a lowly hand surgeon.'

I coughed a laugh. 'She'll be discharged in about a week then?'

'Something like that,' he said. 'I can't say for certain as it all depends on transport and beds. But the nurses on the ward will let you know.'

I was fumbling through the darkness, knowing only darkness lay ahead. The only prick of hope was that the doctors were finally in contact. I might not have seen my mother for a year, but I was still her daughter.

Chapter Forty-Eight

Elinor's Prognosis

Hi Helen, I've been visiting my grandad in hospital and your mum's here. Did you know? love Carys x

I wasn't aware she'd been discharged from Birmingham. In fact, if it wasn't for Carys's text message, I wouldn't have had any idea Mum had been moved. After all that contact, all those times the doctors rang me wanting information, I thought they might bother to call when Mum was discharged. But after I got the text from Carys – when I rang the ward, the matron, the doctor, the consultant – my calls went unanswered. The only way of getting a response was by making a complaint. My strength was being sucked out.

'I'm sorry, it was an absolute oversight,' the matron in Birmingham said. It was amazing how quickly she'd responded once my complaint had been made.

'I want to know why it's happened,' I demanded. 'I am her only daughter, the only relative.'

'I understand that, and I can only apologise. We contacted her next of kin—'

'I am her next of kin.'

'Yes, I understand that. But on her medical notes it's down as Mrs Annette Wright.'

I put down the phone and growled into the air, listening as it reverberated through the empty house. I stabbed the number for Mum's local hospital into my mobile and repeated the same conversation with the matron on my mother's ward.

'Did Elinor request for Mrs Wright to be noted as next of kin?' I asked, my hands trembling.

'Your mother's in no fit state to request anything,' matron said.

'It needs to be changed right now,' I said, my fingers frozen and white around my mobile. 'I am the next of kin. I am to be informed – not a friend, not anyone else.'

My outrage was forcing me outside my body to witness this assertive version of myself. I was certain I wasn't being unreasonable, certain that, despite everything, they should have contacted me instead of Annette. I might not be there, but that didn't mean I didn't care or wasn't important. I insisted I speak to the consultant immediately and, for once, I was put through.

'She's been discharged,' the consultant said with disinterest, audibly flicking through paperwork. 'The experts are in Birmingham. There's nothing more for us to do here. We're preparing for her to go to a nursing home.'

'But what's wrong with her?' I demanded, storming up and down the kitchen. I wanted a diagnosis to explain why this was happening, be it physical or – more likely – psychological. 'She's bed bound, incontinent, bent up, barely eating, confused—'

'All I know is she's been discharged,' he interrupted, closing her medical notes loudly. 'There's nothing more to be done.'

There was a dent in my forehead from where I'd been banging my head on a brick wall for four years, and this doctor certainly wasn't going to change the established order. Only the Consultant Neurologist, Dr Froome, could explain why a patient who was deteriorating was being discharged without explanation. His inability to be contacted was exacerbated by his tenure in two hospitals, with separate secretaries running his affairs for each. Although I had contacted the secretaries frequently in both localities, I'd not been allowed Dr Froome's direct number or email, and despite their repeated assurances that he would get back to me, three months had passed without any response. I was so tired of having my life dominated by this black hole.

My letter was short and to the point. I wanted to know what treatment had been carried out. I wanted to know what the results were. I wanted to know what the diagnosis was. I wanted to know if he thought Elinor was going to die; and if so, what was going to kill her. It was my last hope to understand what was happening.

I sent it to both secretaries by registered post.

I sent it to both secretaries by email.

Four copies of the same letter, which were followed by two weeks of silence.

I sent it to both secretaries again by registered post.

I sent it to both secretaries again by email.

I sent it to Dr Froome via both hospitals' Patient Advice and Liaison Service (PALS) offices.

That's ten copies and two more weeks of silence.

I contacted both PALS offices again to say that I would be making a formal complaint.

I received Dr Froome's letter the next day.

Chapter Forty-Nine

A Difficult Diagnosis

Dr Michael Froome
Consultant Neurologist
1st July 2016
RE: Elinor Page

I must apologise for the delay but I needed time to get hold of the hospital notes.

Prior to me Mrs Page had been under the care of Dr Coldfield, Consultant Psychiatrist, so in answer to your question, the possibility of psychological or psychiatric element to her condition had been addressed. Her admission under my care was primarily to find a reversible structural or chemical problem which unfortunately was not the case.

A multi-disciplinary approach was adopted and she was seen by specialists in rehabilitation medicine, a Consultant Neurologist with a particular interest in movement disorder, a Consultant Orthopaedic Hand Surgeon and a Consultant Gastroenterologist.

There was no evidence of wasting to the brain to suggest a major cognitive neurodegenerative condition such as Alzheimer.

She was weaned off any medication that may exacerbate movement disorders, but no improvement to her rigid state was achieved.

> *As regards to her underlying diagnosis, this is difficult*
> *but she would be clinically described as having an akinetic*
> *rigid syndrome.*
>
> *She does not have straightforward Parkinsonism and does*
> *not respond to the treatment for this.*
>
> *I would have great concerns about her future due to her*
> *difficulty putting on or maintaining weight, her contracture*
> *and potential risk of aspirational pneumonia.*

I re-read the words, hoping they'd make more sense the second time. No physical explanation for her symptoms, a dismissal of any possible psychiatric issues, her future was bleak – and yet she was being discharged.

I doubted I was the first person to listen to endless dial tones, or my mother the first to be given up on. Psychiatric problems are, without question, tangled and briared, but did that mean that it wasn't worth trying to unravel or understand them, as Dr Coldfield, the psychiatrist, had decided? Instead of him delving for an answer, my mother had been left to do whatever she wanted to do – pay for carers she didn't need, go into unnecessary respite care, bind her hands, stop eating – in the name of patient privacy and choice. They'd wasted resources and money on her without question because it was what she wanted and, when she'd deteriorated, she'd been thrown into a system that was only interested in a result that could be quantified – something that could be found in the medical dictionary. And when that wasn't possible, rather than addressing her complex needs, she'd been left to die because she was incapable of making good choices.

As for me, her only family, I'd been ignored as if only the opinions of trained professionals and the patient herself could be worthwhile, all based on the assumption that the patient would tell the truth and make logical decisions. You don't need to be a doctor to know that in every sphere of the health service there are plenty of hypochondriacs, let alone people with more serious mental problems like Munchausen's, who are willing to mislead those there to help them. In retrospect, Mum was displaying a classic case of Munchausen's; when confronted by her Parkinson's nurse, she'd become aggressive, and I could well imagine this had been repeated with others who challenged her.

So, even when it's obvious that these patients aren't physically ill, how can our health services deal with them except to give them what they want, especially if they are antagonised by confrontation?

Dr Froome's letter felt cold and uncompromising, even if he was only following NHS protocol to minimise medical contact. As I later read on the NHS website, since Mum had manipulated, lied and falsified symptoms, 'the patient can no longer be trusted [so] the doctor is unable to continue treating them'. But where does this leave the patient, and the patient's family?

An earlier diagnosis would be possible if doctors were advised to communicate with the patient's family and friends, giving them the bigger picture of the lives of people with Munchausen's. And maybe then, both the health professionals and the patient's families would have more answers, and those mentally ill people wouldn't be left to bounce through the NHS, squandering resources and wreaking havoc on anyone who will believe their lies.

I sat on the bottom stair and re-read the letter. I knew I should have felt furious and appalled that nothing more would be done, spurred on to further complaints and action. I rubbed my eyes until they blurred. I was so tired, my muscles weakened and relenting. I could read between the lines. Dr Froome had searched for a symptom he could treat and had found that nothing more could be done. He'd decided that even psychiatric intervention wouldn't help. It was too late. It was time to give up.

As summer approached, Blossom began pre-school with her turquoise backpack and a big grin, her blonde curls tied back.

Julia told me that Elinor was being treated well in the new nursing home. She was bed bound, being fed, changed and washed by nurses, continuing to bend her joints and becoming permanently frozen in twisted shapes. No longer fed by a tube, her weight was plummeting, she was becoming weaker and she was losing her grip on reality.

I'd become used to seeing the look on people's faces when I said I wasn't going to see my mother again – the shock at my audacity to say the unsayable. I'd heard all the reasons I should go to her bedside – I didn't want our relationship to end badly; I'd regret it; I needed to make amends; I shouldn't judge Elinor on her last few years – but they were all based on the assumption that my mother was normal and our relationship had, at some point, been healthy.

Whatever version of a final encounter with my mother I envisioned, it involved the truth being manipulated and distorted, leaving me tortured by shame. My mother wasn't normal: she didn't want the best for me, she didn't care for my needs and she wasn't good. For my mother, an ending where I was crushed would be the very best outcome.

Chapter Fifty

Letting Go

Though summer was drifting away, the days were warm, the sunlight catching the luscious green of the garden and making me nostalgic. I was painfully conscious that the season would soon turn, the leaves would brown and curl, the sun would drop low in the sky and I would have to dig out my big coat. Bailey had started Year One and, since Blossom was at pre-school, I had two precious hours a day when I could enjoy dawdling in the supermarket, drinking coffee and talking to adults without interruption.

Joy and I sat in my lounge, curled up to face each other on the sofa. A friend of a friend, with a background in psychiatry, she had blown into my life at the right moment. A petite woman, her clothes were utilitarian, her salt-and-pepper hair cut short for ease. Though she didn't fidget, she had an energy about her that made me think she rarely relaxed.

'I know you can't give me the definitive truth of what's going on,' I said, clasping a cappuccino, 'but I want some informed ideas. I think she's got a personality disorder.'

She tilted her head. 'What about her parents, her family? Any history of illnesses?'

'They're all hypochondriacs,' I said. 'Her father was a pharmacist. Her grandmother took to bed for twenty years for no apparent reason.'

'Personality disorders are difficult things,' she said. 'They're nice, neat labels, but life is rarely like that. What about her childhood?'

'She said she was the underdog in her family,' I said, 'She was like her father. Her mother said she would be a career woman and so she tried to prove she could have a family too. She married Dad and her whole life revolved around work – she loved her job, and all her friends were there. But then they had me, and that all ended. Dad got ill, Mum's ME followed and it dominated our lives.'

Joy drank her tea slowly, gazing into middle distance while I stayed mute.

'This could be one suggestion,' she said finally, putting down her cup. 'Say your mum was brought up in a household where she felt ignored. She holds her father in high regard – he's the epitome of success for her – and this is reinforced by her mother saying that Elinor is like him. But he's out of the house a lot, and Elinor grows up in this environment where she feels disregarded and 'otherly'. She's wanting and failing to get her father's love. And she learns, from her grandmother, as well as her father's profession, that when you are ill you get a lot of attention and care.

'Then along comes your dad. Maybe she doesn't know what love is. She's a shell of a person, imitating what she thinks she should be. Your dad keeps her afloat and she builds this successful life in her workplace. But then she makes this terrible mistake and has a baby. Because when her mother said she was a career woman, she was right. The identity that she's managed to create at work is lost and underneath there isn't anything.

'Your dad gets ill, and it reminds her that when you are unwell you get a lot of care. She stumbles across ME – the 'Yuppy Flu' was all over the news at that time – and it's perfect. There's no tests, no treatment, no medical intervention. It's the perfect hiding place for someone pretending to be ill. It becomes who she is – her new identity. And it gives her a lot of attention and a lot of success – she's practically running the local ME group, single-handedly producing the newsletter, hailed as Local Health Champion. A very successful ill person. Lots of praise and recognition, all the stamps of approval to show everyone she's disabled. I would imagine whenever the attention starts to wane, she can have a relapse. And those who don't believe she's unwell have to be cut off because otherwise she might be exposed. It's a dangerous tightrope.

'It's not that she didn't love you as such, if she ever had any idea what love was. It was that preserving her identity was far more important. She obviously loved you, otherwise she wouldn't have sought your attention or put so much effort into manipulating you.'

'I don't get it though,' I said, when Joy fell quiet. 'If she loved me and my dad so much, why, after he died, did she go round destroying everything? Cutting off her wedding rings?'

Joy stopped and looked at the ceiling thoughtfully before turning back to me. 'Perhaps she was punishing him. He'd let her down, like her father had. Abandoned her. You said she started talking about the power of attorney after your dad died? Maybe she was hoping she'd die too.'

'But she had this new identity of widow. Wasn't that enough?'

'That's only a short-term plan for attention though, isn't it?' she said with a sarcastic tut. 'She needs something else. Something bigger. Your dad's last few years – all those emergency dashes to hospital and the constant flow of doctors – might have tarnished her success with the ME. Plus, you'd abandoned her by having children. Obviously,' Joy said, touching my knee lightly, 'I'm saying this is how your mother might have been viewing events. It's perfectly natural to care for your children. But from her point of view, they were her new rivals for attention. She needed to ramp it up to get you back.'

'Ah,' I said. 'so, the Parkinson's.'

Joy chuckled. 'In a way it was her biggest mistake. ME was ideal because she didn't need to prove anything and the doctors just accepted she's disabled. But when she chose Parkinson's Disease, for whatever reason…'

'Her father had Benign Essential Tremor,' I added. 'A shaking of his hands.'

'A link to her father,' Joy said, nodding. 'Imitating him perhaps. But with Parkinson's she couldn't make it up. There are specific, identifiable symptoms. From the outside that must have made it very attractive to your mum: all the nurses, doctors and medication. But ultimately it's a dead end because they're actually assessing you and they can tell if you don't act the symptoms out correctly. You can't just say you have dystonia and make it true by the force of your own will.'

I shuffled around the sofa. 'I don't understand why she keeps going with it though. Doesn't it ruin it that we all know she's making it up?'

Joy didn't miss a beat. 'She's been so successful with the ME that she might think you'll believe her if she keeps going. Perhaps she is compelled. At some point you cross over from controlling an addiction to being controlled. And the idea of choice is interesting. She probably didn't have as many choices as you think she did. Without the disabled label she doesn't have anything. Beneath the pretence, psychologically speaking, she doesn't have an identity.'

I felt my throat tightening. 'That makes me feel so sad.'

She calmly passed me a tissue from her bag, dropping her voice to a gentle lull as I dabbed my face. 'It doesn't change anything though. She'll continue to drag you into it and manipulate you because that's all she's got. Ultimately she wants you to sacrifice your children and your life to care for her. That's not healthy for any of you.' She sought my eye and reached out a hand. 'But perhaps having an idea of why she's doing it makes it easier to forgive her.'

She took up her tea and sat back on the sofa, cradling the lukewarm mug in her hands. 'It's a shame because if she'd have carried on with the ME, she could have lived her life that way. No one would have questioned it, there would've been lots of attention, you'd still be caring for her, we wouldn't be having this conversation. She could've had quite a good end to her life. I mean, it would've been a lie, but you wouldn't have known that, and she was happy in her little fiction. Choosing Parkinson's has blown that all up. She's had to go to extremes. She must be very tortured, inside and out.'

'Do you think,' I said, hacking the words out from my dry throat, 'that I could've done anything? I've tried to speak to her doctors and consultants, but most of them wouldn't even acknowledge me.'

Joy grasped my hand again. 'No one could've done anything. Perhaps when she first started pretending to have ME, if a doctor had really questioned her and referred her to the right psychiatrist. But then, it wasn't clear, was it? And you said there were family and friends who stood up to her at that time and she cut them off. She wasn't going to listen.

'By the time it was obvious, it was too late. Even if Dr Coldfield had decided to do something, it probably wouldn't have got her anywhere. She was too far down the road by then, let alone now. And you've done everything you can. You have tried to save her and now you're honouring her decision. You have to care for yourself and your family.'

Once Joy had left, the house was quiet and dark with shadows. I sat on the sofa and cried but not out of desperation any more. I was so sad for my mother's wasted life. Everything had changed and so had nothing. I knew I had to forgive her. If I tried to hold onto the hurt, it would bind me to my mother and, even though she would never apologise, I needed to be free of her grip on me.

I didn't believe my mother had been unable to choose to do good. She'd been wise enough to use the secret moments, when no one else was around, to destroy me; that wasn't desperate but devious. Still, Joy had given me a starting point to practise forgiveness, something I would repeat relentlessly. It allowed me to let my mother go.

Chapter Fifty-One

Phone Call

The wind was howling as we walked to school the next day, the dust and leaves rising up in smoky gusts that stung my eyes. I held the children's hands tightly and pulled them into the twitchel where we'd be sheltered from the worst of it.

'Crikey,' I said. 'I'm glad we came this way.'

'I can hear you again, Mummy,' Bailey said, pulling down the hood on his Batman coat and letting go of my hand.

'You won't get blown away now,' I laughed as he raced down the alleyway, Blossom in pursuit, spinning as if they were tornadoes.

It wasn't often that my phone rang at eight thirty on a Tuesday morning. I scrambled to pull my mobile out of my pocket and to my ear.

'This is Mrs Page's nursing home.'

I was instantly shaking as if I'd had too much caffeine, my insides whizzing around like the children down the cut through. Was this it? All these months I'd been waiting in the cold of no man's land, uncertain if I'd even be informed when she died. I was too hot, even in the biting wind.

'I'm calling to let you know your mother has got a mouth infection,' the woman said with stiff formality. They hadn't called me when Elinor had a chest infection – I'd found out from Julia – so why were they were calling me now? 'She's been given antibiotics and the doctor is coming back to see her in a week.'

I knew I was party to a coded conversation, one for which I didn't have the key. 'Okay,' I said, the school gates coming into view ahead of us. 'Will you let me know what he says next week then?'

The pause was too long, the woman clearly confounded by my response.

'Well… she is very weak.'

'Okay,' I said, hoping my drawn-out words might force her to say more. 'Will you call me in a couple of days then?'

'Yes, okay. Or sooner.'

It wasn't obvious. Nothing told me definitively what was happening, and I didn't know what to do with the information. I put my phone back in my pocket and ran after the children, the school bell ringing ahead of us.

'You alright?' Jemma said. 'You're usually early.'

'Had a strange phone call,' I said, as I waved Bailey into his class. 'About my mum.'

We turned and walked away in the throng of other parents, like water pouring out of the gate and down the street.

'I don't know what it means. Could be the end or could be nothing.'

Jemma gave me a hug. 'Let's go for coffee.'

The conversation simmered in the back of my mind that day and, like a song on loop that I couldn't forget, it interrupted my sleep.

I didn't often let Bailey play on the slide in the pre-school playground while I took Blossom into nursery, but the next day I relented. Blossom proudly hung her bag on the hook with her photo and led me through the jam of parents and carers. She found her picture on a rubber band, chose which milk carton she wanted and labelled it easily while the other children struggled – a small skill that made me unduly proud. She was about to go into her classroom when I felt my mobile buzzing. I knew who it was and why they were calling, but phones were not allowed in school. I was hyper aware, panicking and trying not to panic, knowing I wouldn't be able to get to Bailey. I kissed Blossom mechanically. The room was too full, and I couldn't get out, my phone vibrating urgently. Pushing through I burst into the sunlight, finding Jemma before I could see Bailey.

'Are you okay?'

'I've got to take a call.'

'Okay,' she said, and she knew. 'I've got Bailey.'

I marched out of the gates, fumbling to redial the number and thinking how useless I'd be in an emergency. It rang twice before someone answered. The nurse's voice was serious straight away.

'I'm afraid your mother has taken a turn for the worst.'

I felt a rush of anger, a sweeping panic. I was back to the hospital where Dad had died, back to the uncertainty of euphemisms and nauseating fear. I couldn't see straight or hear properly because of the thumping in my ears. I leant back heavily on the school gate in the hope that it would hold me up.

'In what way?'

I had to hear her say the words, to tell me the day I'd been longing for and dreading had arrived. My legs began to wobble, my brain overheating; I could barely hear the answer.

'I'm afraid she's passed away.'

I slumped to the ground. 'W-when did she go?'

The school bell had rung, and parents were passing me by as they headed out into their day, free from children. I wiped my make-up across my face and didn't care that they were staring at me.

'About half an hour ago,' she said, and I checked my watch so I knew what time Mum had gone.

'And… w-what happens now?'

'Oh!' she said. 'Well, you contact a funeral director and then get back in touch with us.'

I was a thirty-year-old orphan, but was that a thing? Do you stop being an orphan after you reach eighteen, or does it count even if you're seventy? There was no other family, I was the only one left and I felt like I was sixteen. I didn't know what you said to a funeral director or the proper way to meet a solicitor or how to be an executor. Thirty-something adults are supposed to be able to deal with these things, but I felt adrift. I wanted my mum.

'And… and her things, what happens with them?'

'Don't worry, they're here,' she said in a kinder voice, finally realising I was in shock. 'Call us back when you're ready. I'm so sorry for your loss.'

I laid my head in my hands, letting them take on large mascara stigmata, before pulling myself up and stumbling back to the playground. I fell into Jemma's arms.

'I don't know what to do,' I said in large, ugly sobs.

'Call Peter.'

'But… there's no reason for him to come home, is there? There's nothing to do.'

'Yeah,' she said, unconvinced. 'You need to call Peter.'

I thought I might have lost my mind entirely. I called Peter and told him he didn't need to come home and, despite Jemma's offer of a lift, I decided to walk. I dragged myself the quarter of a mile to my house as Peter pulled up outside. As he wrapped his arms around me, I took my first breath since I spoke to the nurse. Inside, I sat on the sofa and noted the time. It was 9.10 a.m. One hour earlier my mother had died.

Chapter Fifty-Two

Funeral

For days I didn't exist. Peter did the school run and the food shopping, the cleaning and the cooking, the phone calls and the arrangements. He kept life running while I failed to participate, floating around the house like an apparition and teetering on matchstick stilts when I tentatively ventured outside, one step away from total collapse.

'I need to tell you something.'

The last faint fireworks of summer had been replaced by dull, grey apathy that closeted the house. I was watching TV, masking my emotions with something that didn't require anything of me. I looked up at Peter and knew.

'It's Annette, isn't it?'

I'd suspected for months that something wasn't right, ever since Annette had stopped contacting me. While Julia, Sandy and Judy had been increasingly supportive, especially since Dr Froome's letter, Annette's silence had become a lurking shadow. Though she ignored my emails, I was told she continued to pop into the flat at the Lilly Fields regularly with her own key. When Peter had informed her of Elinor's death, asking her to keep it to herself while we told my relatives, she'd given a terse reply. And then, the day after Mum died, I'd called the nursing home to arrange for Julia to collect my mother's belongings.

'It's alright,' said the nurse. 'One of Elinor's friends is coming this afternoon.'

'What? Who's picking them up?' I said, already knowing the answer.

'Annette Wright.'

'No,' I said, my heart rate rising. 'No, I don't want Annette to collect them. I'll arrange for someone to come.'

I sent Annette a text message.

Julia is going to pick up my mum's belongings, thanks. As you've already started telling people the news please can you inform them it will be a private funeral.

I'd decided many months before that my mother's funeral would be a small, intimate gathering. I couldn't face crowds of people telling me how Elinor would be missed, how greatly they loved her, how sorry they were for my loss. It was hard enough reading the sympathy cards that had started to arrive, messages full of regard for my mother's kindness, generosity and loveliness. She may have convinced some people that she was good, but undoubtedly Mum was playing them. If only they knew what she'd said about them behind closed doors. She'd made a fool of all of us, and I didn't want to stand in a room of my mother's lies. I wanted to be honest because my complicated grief was more important than my duty towards any distant family members, or friends who had been duped into enabling my mother. Annette did not reply to my text message.

Peter flinched as I said her name. He sat beside me and took my hand. 'Yeah, it's about Annette. Julia went to pick up the key to the Lilly Fields flat. Annette asked her in, sat Julia down, and then she and her husband started laying into you. They told Julia what a bad daughter you are because you didn't visit your mum. Annette is furious about the private funeral and that she's not going to be there.'

'She was going to be invited.'

'Yeah, but she didn't know that, did she?' Peter said, raising his eyebrows. 'She told Julia she's going to turn up at the funeral and "give you a piece of her mind" so everyone will know what you've done. But at least she's given Julia the key.'

'That must have been terrifying. Poor Julia.' I put my head into my hands. 'This is all my fault.' I could feel the last drops of energy seeping out of my arms and legs.

'This is not your fault,' Peter said, pulling me into his chest. 'Not even slightly! We knew something funny was going on, didn't we?'

I rubbed my face vigorously in the hope I would wipe the fog from my head. 'It's interesting that she jumped to the conclusion she's not invited to the funeral. She was top of the list.'

'She *was*!' Peter scoffed. 'We can't invite her now.'

I let out a heavy breath and scrubbed at my face. 'If I hadn't sent her that message, we wouldn't have known what she was planning. She would have turned up – probably with her husband and her sons – and shouted at me in front of everyone.'

I was too broken to cry any more. I couldn't understand what was driving Annette's behaviour. I didn't know what she wanted from me. Only in soap operas would someone turn up to a funeral to give those grieving a piece of their mind. It wasn't proportional. It was more exaggerated drama.

'You know there was nothing more you could've done,' Peter said. 'If Annette wanted to sacrifice her life while your mum destroyed herself, then that's her choice, but she's no right to say you should do the same. It was an impossible situation.'

I was blown along by the momentum of events. My feet didn't touch the ground as Peter and I travelled to my home town while the children stayed with Jemma for their first night away from us. We spent the day searching Mum's flat for the necessary documents to arrange her funeral, digging through the avalanche of boxes in the second bedroom.

The organised chaos of paperwork covered her whole life: the details regarding the sale of their house in the 1970s; every letter her schoolfriend had sent her since they were twelve; the receipts for every large purchase she'd made in her life. The recognisable objects from my childhood were lifeless, an accumulated jumble that hadn't settled into its new environment. I struggled to understand why my mother had chosen to bring these items to her new flat – a broken ornate clock, four outdated mobile phones, a box of 1950s glass Christmas decorations – but not her wedding dress. She'd kept every birthday card she'd ever received but not that long-sleeved, high-necked, white lace gown. Had these items been chosen specifically? Or were they brought here accidentally, hidden amongst more desirable items? I was hysterical, feeling the pressure of finding the papers we required in the limited time available, unable to stop my panicked laughter. I wasn't really there; I was only an outline of what I needed to be.

When we'd found what we needed, we retreated back to Julia's to drink heavily dosed gin and tonics. Julia's cottage was lit with candles, the fire crackling soothingly as we lay on her soft, cream sofa, snuggled amongst blankets and cushions.

'It's probably going to say multiple organ failure,' Julia said as she passed me the envelope. A formal brown A4, it might well have contained A-level results rather than a death certificate. I put my hands up defensively.

'Can you open it?'

I was a heady mixture of exhaustion and manic alertness, as if the lights were too bright for me to see properly. Julia slid a finger through the seal, pulling jagged, awkward sections.

'Oh,' she said as she read it. Peter edged forward on the armchair in anticipation. 'I suppose we can say she got what she wanted. "Cause of Death: Parkinson's Disease".'

My breath was being sucked out of me. 'How could they say that?' I said. 'She'd been taken off all the meds in Birmingham, checked for even the weird types of Parkinson's.'

'You don't die of Parkinson's anyway,' Peter said, falling back into the chair. 'You die from symptoms caused by Parkinson's.'

'Quite,' Julia said, brushing a wayward ringlet from her face. 'I'm amazed they've chosen to put this. I would guess the doctor read her medical notes, saw she'd been on Parkinson's medication, assessed that she's got these contractures and so forth and that's what he's gone with.'

'It's so lazy,' I said, balling my hands up.

'It says something though, doesn't it?' Peter said. 'About the power of the mind. She absolutely wanted to die of Parkinson's and that's what her death certificate says.'

I swallowed down some more gin, feeling the hole in my chest widen. After everything – all the tests, all the proof – she'd won. It would go down in history that she died of Parkinson's, the truth remaining hidden in shadows.

'What *did* she die of then?' I said, leaning on Julia's shoulder.

'She would have been so weak in her malnourished state, and from not moving for so long, that she would have got that little mouth infection – one that you and I could easily fight off – and it would have been too much for her body to take.'

Peter moved onto the sofa and put his arm around me. My face was streaked and salty. 'It's such a sad end.'

'I know, darling,' Julia said.

It was cold but bright on the day of her funeral, the season falling fully into autumn's embrace. I'd spent the morning in the toilet, the true meaning of shitting yourself realised. Julia's adult children intended to guard the crematorium door and the funeral director had been strictly advised not to advertise the event. But my imagination ran wild with visions of Annette, her towering husband and her huge sons bursting in with furious accusations.

A dramatic send-off might have been more appropriate, but Mum's funeral comprised two rows of chosen guests and no inter-ruptions. Apart from my second cousin Owain, who sent me an angry email berating me for leaving out the 'closest relatives', though neither my mother nor I had seen or heard from him in years, my extended family was generally understanding – if somewhat mystified – by my choice of a private funeral. And I was single minded in believing that only in private would I be able to be honest, determined to have a chance to cry my own complicated tears for the mum I had lost and the mum I had wanted her to be.

It feels uncomfortable now to see myself controlling the story, defending my version of events and my image of Elinor. Just like Mum did, I was preserving my truth, framing it with people who agreed with me. The similarities make me squirm, but it wasn't a case of bending the truth – rather allowing myself to mourn freely when no one else appeared to want to grieve. Annette had made it clear she intended to use the funeral to rail against my lack of contact with Mum in her final months. For my cousin Owain, attending the funeral was about recognition. It was his blood right to be there, and I owed him the deference. And for my wider family, most of whom hadn't had contact with my mother since she went into the care home, their attendance would have been out of duty, not to grieve. These distant family members – as well as Mum's long-lost friends, the ME group, and others who might have come to the service – only knew a part of what had happened. I couldn't bear for them to tell me how wonderful Mum was – how loved, how missed – when I knew what she'd really been, and I knew what she'd said about these same people behind their backs. She'd deviously used them, even if they didn't realise, and I couldn't mentally handle their misplaced platitudes. It was self-preservation. But then, Mum's actions – the endless manipulation and shaping of events, holding others at a distance and culling those who didn't agree with her story – was also a form of self-preservation.

I can't deny that there are regular similarities in our lives. It's only the reasons behind our actions that separate us, and even then, it's complex. Mum constantly put herself, her desires and her truth first, but to be the opposite of her doesn't mean I should never put myself first. The opposite is that I prioritise myself when I genuinely need to practise self-care, and sometimes that will mean my behaviour and reasoning will overlap with Mum's, even if I'm not being selfish. It's a tension I struggle with, a parallel I hate to draw.

'Perhaps,' I said, as we ate cake afterwards, the tension and tears drained into muted quiet, 'I could quote Spike Milligan's epitaph on her gravestone.'

'*I told you I was ill?*' Julia said, breaking into laughter.

'Even more ironic, don't you think?' I said, wiping my face.

I'd had quite enough of wearing a facade to make other people feel better. At my mother's funeral I had finally been honest.

Chapter Fifty-Three

Rings

All four of us were crammed into Julia's little cottage for the longest short weekend, with too much to achieve and not enough time. I was all too aware that our presence had broken the house's usual calm, the large, white cushion of a cat staring daggers at me as we ate breakfast together.

'Tell me, darling, are we doing the jewellers first?' Julia asked, holding her granary toast, slathered in butter, mid-air. Blossom was tracing the embroidered dragonflies on Julia's shirt, pushing her purple cardigan out of the way so she could discover further insects.

'Yes,' I said, pouring milk onto Bailey's cornflakes. 'I don't know why, but I have a feeling we need to get them urgently.'

'They couldn't be any safer,' Peter said, rolling his eyes.

I dropped my head to my shoulder, 'I know.'

'Do you know how many there are?' Julia asked.

'Three,' I said. 'Wedding ring, engagement ring and eternity ring. All cut into pieces. Going to be easily identifiable.'

'I'll meet you at your mum's flat,' Peter said with a weary glance at the children who were still in their pyjamas. 'When we eventually get there.'

I gripped onto Julia's arm as we walked from the car park, the death certificate burning hot in my bag. Even two weeks after her death, I was unsteady on my feet, the very thought of retrieving the rings exhausting me. The door was weighted, the narrow corridor of a shop shadowed by wooden panelling, as if the owners were trying to dissuade anyone from entering. A long glass counter ran down the centre, dividing customer from staff, filled with treasures that sparkled between us. The jeweller was a tall, thin man with small, half-moon glasses that sat on his long nose. He shuffled awkwardly from foot to foot and massaged his chin.

'The thing is, you don't have the receipt.'

'We've searched her flat,' I said. 'But we can't find it. I can describe the rings if that's helpful.'

He pored over the death certificate again as if it might give him extra clues. 'No, this will do,' he said, turning on his heels and heading into the back of the shop, letting the hefty door close behind him.

'I didn't think he was going to let us have them,' Julia said. 'He's very cautious.'

'Isn't he?' I said, peering at the gold bands inside the counter. 'He said on the phone that the death certificate would be enough.'

The door to the back of the shop swung open and the jeweller re-emerged carrying a tiny, black coffin, holding it closely as he approached us.

'I'm uneasy,' he said, pulling a nervous half-smile. 'You see, we had another lady in here a couple of days ago asking for the same rings.'

I felt like I'd been winded, but Julia was impressively breezy.

'Oh really?' she said. 'I don't suppose she had short pink hair?'

'That's the one,' he said.

Julia and I swapped heavy looks, but our reactions seemed to relieve the jeweller who stepped forward, his face relaxing.

'She was quite insistent,' he continued. 'Said they were her deceased friend's but she'd lost the receipt. I told her, as I told you, that she needed the death certificate. She didn't take that well. Rather pushy in fact, which, in my job, suggests a problem.'

'I imagine good instincts are essential in your job,' Julia said, sharing a smile with him.

'Indeed. You know they're broken?'

'Yes,' I said. 'She had them cut off.'

'That's right,' he said, passing me the little box.

I turned it over in my hands. It would be several years before I was able to look at the tarnished lumps of metal that had once been displayed with such pride on my mother's long, slender fingers.

We arrived home on Sunday night, the long drive extended by lashing, autumnal rain and utter exhaustion. The children raced off to their bedrooms, eager to reacquaint themselves with their toys, as we dragged in our suitcases. I picked up a pristine, white envelope from the doormat, my hair sticking to my face. Our address was typed incorrectly onto a label and inside was a ripped photocopy of the local newspaper. There was no accompanying note.

LOSS FOR M.E. GROUP

Elinor Page recently passed away. She was wonderful and kind. She helped so many people with M.E.. She worked at the M.E. group for years and she was the secretary and treasurer. Elinor had M.E. and later Parkinson's. She became very ill and had to give up working for the group. We all loved her and thanked her for her hard work. Rest in peace and God bless you.

From all of her friends at the M.E. group.

The group meets in the community hall next to Woolworths every fourth Thursday of the month at 3:15. Everyone is welcome. Contact details below.

I felt furious, as if my veins were pumping with burning magma. It didn't seem like a respectful tribute; they were using my mother's death as an advertisement for their group. Sending it to me, like this – on a torn-off piece of paper, without a condolence card or letter – didn't feel like an act of sympathy. It was either a poor afterthought or a disapproving gesture.

How did my mother have this power over others? I'd hoped that once she was gone the drama would be finished, but still I was dealing with Elinor's friends threatening to storm the funeral, writing obituaries and visiting the jewellers without my permission. They were such drastic measures, and I didn't understand why they thought it was appropriate.

Annette would go on to arrange and pay for a memorial service for Elinor a few months later. She booked out an entire pub in readiness for a crowd and contacted many of my mother's acquaintances, the ME group and some of my distant family – mostly people who hadn't seen or heard from Elinor in years. I was told that, despite her efforts, only a handful of mourners attended, sharing scattered memories and reassembling a good life from the stories Elinor had told them. Perhaps they believed that recalling her tales would exonerate Elinor's last years, but to me it only reinforced how conniving she was. Her manipulations had always relied on our unquestioning devotion and, from beyond the grave, she continued to control the narrative.

I still wonder what caused these few devoted admirers to go to such lengths. They may have been driven by grief, though their extreme and secretive actions didn't suggest that to me. I could more readily believe that they just couldn't accept that Elinor had lied. It was hard for any of us to swallow; Judy was furious, Julia shocked, Sandy heartbroken. This woman, who'd appeared so vulnerable, weak and pathetic, had lied and schemed to make us sacrifice ourselves for her. We'd held her arm as she walked, done her shopping, driven her places, pushed her in a wheelchair, cleared her house and, all the time, she was perfectly well and able. It was humiliating.

While others had backed away from Elinor's lies, perhaps Annette felt she had no choice but to collaborate, believing Elinor because she'd put so much time, energy and trust into their relationship. Elinor had made it clear that Annette must either choose to believe her or be cut off. So Annette had continued to care for Elinor, believing she was helping her and leaving no room for an alternative; I had to be the problem in the situation and she was still determined to prove it.

For the ME group the revelation would have been devastating. Admitting that their secretary, treasurer and Local Health Champion had been making it up the whole time would create unimaginable damage to their cause. It was much easier to make out that I was abusing my mother's memory and denying their grief than to accept Elinor faked it all.

I felt like I was met with anger and disgust at every turn because I hadn't been in contact with Elinor at the end. My grief was complex, but it was still grief. I wished things had been different. I wished I could have reconciled with my mother before she died. I wished she'd been the mother I wanted her to be. I'd loved my mum, even more than her friends and acquaintances had, and the truth was life-shattering agony. But for me there was nothing to gain from denying it any more.

Chapter Fifty-Four

The Diaries

I remember there was a day, many months after my mother had died, when I realised I hadn't cried for a whole week. It was a revelation after the insanity of the previous years. Life was much easier without my mother around. No longer thrown between contrasting worlds of light and dark, I could finally concentrate on my family.

The first September since my mother's death, Blossom started in Reception, her purple gingham school dress tickling the tops of her calves. Jemma and I joked we'd become ladies who lunched, but the idea of solely housekeeping was too close to Mum's life. I dreaded becoming her, but, since Mum had trained me to see any self-care as laziness and failure, I wasn't going to copy her anyway.

Since I was a child, I'd loved to write stories, plays, poems and songs. I'd created characters and adventures and loved seeing the words form on a page. Now I had the opportunity to focus on writing and I had a bizarre story to tell. The words were bubbling up within me, my fingers itchy to type. But I knew, as part of writing it, I'd have to read the diaries.

It took me two years after Mum's death to pluck up the courage to read them. I'd always known the diaries existed, and Mum had happily shared them with me when I was a teen. They hadn't struck me as particularly interesting at the time. When we cleared out Mum's flat, I'd insisted on keeping these tiny books, storing them safely away in my loft, unsure whether I wanted them or not.

When I decided to read them, I began with the last few years of Mum's life – events I could directly compare with my own experiences. I read them in feverish fits punctuated with regular pauses. I felt crushed by the contradictions, the twisted distortions and the outright lies. In the diaries, Elinor made herself the perpetual victim, relaying events in blunt, emotionless stabs. There was no sign of the perfect mother I thought I knew.

I didn't want to read on. And why should I? She'd told me her life story. She'd had a difficult childhood, followed by her golden years in her twenties, which had been ruined by my birth in her thirties. I knew that she'd pretended to have ME through the 1990s and spent all her time in bed faking an illness, but then, in the 2000s, had sacrificially cared for my dad in his final years. What was there to gain from reading her account? Julia told me to throw the diaries away – they were full of lies, she said, and would do me no good. But the weight of them hung on me, the unknown taunting me.

Months later, I resumed reading from the beginning, starting in the 1960s when Elinor was in her early teens. Straight away I was plunged back into Elinor's webbed world, tangled up in her altered perspective. There were days I couldn't see straight – days when the ground wasn't solid and truth was unreachable. I was pummelled by the opposing versions – the stories I'd been told, the diary accounts and my own memories all at odds with each other. Elinor wasn't reliable, but neither was I. My memories bent and faded in the shadow of Elinor's deceit, and no one could console me because no one else had been there. And though I kept taking breaks from the diaries to clear my head, ultimately I had to keep reading. I was wiping away the dirt, clearing the view and hoping that, in the end, I'd be able to see who my mother was.

I'd kept the diaries in a shoe box in my loft. It had once contained a pair of beige, high-heeled Kickers that I'd bought when I was about fourteen, the very height of fashion. Now all that remained of the shoes was the battered box filled with fifty-five tiny pocket diaries. They were all similar sizes, some specifically for schoolgirls, some in lavish gold covers, some with introductory pages of insightful cultural history. In her early diaries Elinor recorded the books she'd taken from the library, while in later ones she'd jotted down text messages she'd received. World events were noted, from Kennedy's assassination and the moon landings through to Thatcher's resignation and onto 9/11. More than five decades of her life squeezed into barely two inches a day, written in her tiny, neat handwriting using varying pens and pencils – the neon green was particularly hard to read. I'd recognise her writing anywhere: the delicate swirls of her z's, her inane misspellings, her characteristic turns of phrase.

Even from the beginning the diaries show aspects of her character that could easily classify Elinor as having NPD. She's a vain, self-obsessed and manipulative emotional void. Those first entries aren't written by your typical teenager filled with angst, heartbreak or secrets. Elinor's cold, utilitarian descriptions make it hard to connect to her. Her daily affairs are recorded as factually as the world events, as if she's removed from them. Even when her grandmother dies, she is impassive, describing her parents' grief as foreign concepts viewed from afar. And when her father is rushed to hospital, she describes it without concern: *'Dad started haemorrhaging and Doc sent him straight to hospital. Went to see him and he looks ok. Then I went to Sue's 21st didn't get home till 12. Quite nice.'*

She doesn't mention love either. Alan was her only boyfriend, but her descriptions of meeting, courting and marrying him are disinterested at best. There's no affection, passion or desire for him; and when he proposes, she refuses, writing, *'Said I didn't want to make a mistake.'* The romance is entirely one sided and it feels like Elinor's parents were more enthusiastic and involved in the courtship than she was. That my parents marry at all is bewildering; Alan was obviously determined.

Through the years it becomes apparent that all her relationships are held at arm's length and I notice many of them are conducted on the phone. It's a clever manipulative tool keeping anyone from seeing the full picture. It must have been especially useful when she began to fake the ME. She also makes sure her friends, acquaintances and employees (such as her cleaner, hairdresser and counsellors) are kept in her debt, whether by giving them extravagant presents, loaning money or insisting on paying for meals when they went out. Easily mistakable for generosity, Elinor used this technique to control those around her. You can't confront someone when they're loaning their car to you for free. You can't challenge a person to whom you owe money.

Repeatedly, anyone who questions Elinor is immediately cut off – be that a medical professional, a friend or even her family. These 'persecutors' are met with classic narcissistic rage – explosions of fury and vitriol when Elinor doesn't get her own way. Throughout the diaries Elinor twists the truth to make herself the victim: her friend is blinded by jealousy; her parents are abusive and cruel; her doctors are ill informed and prejudiced. It makes sense of why her friends and Alan put up with her illogical behaviour. As I did, they too must have known – even subconsciously – that if you didn't stick to Elinor's version of events, then she would leave you.

Though she was never assessed or diagnosed with Munchausen's, it's easy to spot it in the diaries; her obsession with illness is there from the start. Every cold is flu, every temperature is life threatening, and the doctor is called out for a headache. There are constant minor issues – fainting episodes, lists of allergies and strange falls – even when she's a young, healthy woman. And throughout the fifty-five years she has mysterious symptoms that, despite tests and referrals, are never explained. Always leaping to the worst-case scenario, spread over the years she moans of having glandular fever twice, a blood clot in her foot, a detached retina, a trapped nerve, a prolapse, an abscess, IBS, tennis elbow, MSG poisoning, sprained vertebrae and swine flu amongst many other health issues; but none of these problems are confirmed by doctors. She goes for kidney, bone, brain and breast scans, endless x-rays and blood tests, all of which come back clear, yet her GP still refers her on for every complaint. Even standard menopausal symptoms get her sent to a consultant and I can almost hear the doctor's sigh when he sees Mrs Page has another appointment. She must have been a nightmare patient, but her requests for referrals were almost always conceded and she doesn't record any mental health assessments. Yet, amongst all this hypochondria, there's no hint of Elinor fretting about her health. Instead she delights in illness and is disappointed when tests return negative.

In the 1980s it feels as if she's searching for an illness to claim. She notes an address in the back of her 1986 diary, adding, '*For info about cancer, drugs, treatment*', and writes of her titillation at attending a talk on the same subject, though no one she knew had cancer in the surrounding years. In the late 1980s there's a couple of occasions where she writes, '*Helen didn't go to school because I was too ill to take her.*' She describes leaving me, aged six, to do the housework while she went to bed – something uncharacteristic which I don't remember doing – but later that day, when Dad gets home from work, we go to the Beefeater for dinner. I was caring for her even before the ME charade began. No wonder I felt like I was responsible for her.

Her ME appears with a flash in 1991. The first hint she was unwell is denoted by a sentence: '*Sat down in pm and read about "my" illness.*' Within a month she had a diagnosis of ME from the doctor, was '*buying up*' health food shops and taking her temperature daily, though it's always normal. A month after that she was designated a disabled parking badge and was soon using a stick. Rapidly, she embraced this new version of vanity, shedding her fashionable clothes and morphing into a vulnerable, disabled woman who dressed and acted decades older than her years. It was an exhilarating new identity, and successful deception clearly gave her a narcissistic buzz. Her trilling descriptions of being charged for an OAP lunch though she was only in her fifties or having a cleaner who was older than she was are uncomfortable to read, but her outright celebrations when ME hit the news make me shiver: '*News – ME is serious illness like MS and MD! Exciting.*'

Still, none of this was a surprise to me. I knew being ill was an addiction that absorbed Elinor entirely. ME was her favourite topic, and she was vocal about how the ME impacted her life – the many hours in bed, the few short trips she was able to make around town bookended by week-long rests. So to find in the diaries that Elinor's life continued as normal and that she didn't even try to play the part was cataclysmic.

She didn't take daily rests, instead going shopping or socialising every single day. It was the life of a normal, healthy woman – the total opposite to the life Elinor said she lived. While I was at school, she and Dad regularly went apple picking and took day trips to the nearest cities, several hours away from home. There are plenty of occasions when I would have seen her behaving normally, like our annual non-stop holidays where Elinor didn't rest and didn't mention being in pain. It staggers me how normal her life was, how unaffected she was by her 'disability', and yet I continued to believe she was disabled. My eyes are painfully wide open now: her deception was in plain sight.

Even by her own categorisation, Elinor's ME is a fraud. In 1992, her second year of ME, she colour codes her daily diary entries – blue for bad, yellow for '*lots of rest to achieve the minimum*' and pink for '*either did something spectacular like food shopping without (too much) resulting pain or exhaustion or pottering day with less than 4 hours rest*'. Her pink days are coincidentally timed – her birthday, hair appointments and evenings out with friends all fall on these days – but she doesn't stick to these pigeon holes, instead doing multiple activities on a blue day and having pink days after a busy week. She can act spontaneously too, having the spare energy to drop everything and go to a new shop when her friend suggests a day out. The only signs in the diaries that she's unwell are her daily self-medicating with alcohol and prescription drugs and her complaints of feeling awful. She regularly caveats her busy days with '*exhausted*' or '*shattered*', as if being tired after a relentless twenty-four hours isn't normal.

Though it was breathtakingly blatant that Elinor's ME had been a thinly veiled facade, I twisted and turned in my own mind as I read her account, my brain unwilling to accept the deceit. I scolded myself for being too harsh on her. Maybe my memories and her stories and diaries didn't make the whole story. And perhaps I was misjudging ME as an illness. I took for granted that I knew what it looked like after the years of indoctrination from Elinor, but I couldn't trust her version anyway.

According to the NHS, ME symptoms are characterised by an overwhelming and extreme exhaustion but can also include insomnia, muscle pain and flu-like symptoms. Few people are bed bound, but even with the mildest symptoms normal activities are difficult, and sufferers may need to give up work, hobbies or social activities to spend their time resting.

Immediately from this description I can see Elinor doesn't fit. She didn't have extreme exhaustion, her normal activities continued and her daily life didn't alter. Her claims of disability were intentional, malicious lies and she clearly knew what she was doing. There are a couple of occasions where she writes that she '*decided to faint*' and '*decided to get better*', as if it was within her power to be ill or not. It's so obvious from the diaries that she isn't unwell, I don't know how I believed her. Here is naked gaslighting: I instinctively trusted what my mother said and ignored the evidence in front of me. I was just a child and Mum was my bedrock. I believed her entirely. It was more complex for Alan and it's no surprise to find my parents arguing when Elinor refuses to drive or go to social occasions together. Alan wasn't fooled, but he didn't challenge her further.

There's only one time in the diaries when she does seem truly ill, and it has nothing to do with ME. In her typical exaggeration, in 2002 Elinor records she is suffering from '*terrible pain back/ bowel/prolapse*'. The doctor tells her it is a relapse of ME, but Elinor obviously pushes for a referral. After an endoscopy she is diagnosed with duodenitis, and though there is no explanation in the diaries, a quick internet search reveals it is a minor inflammation of the small intestine often caused by long-term use of aspirin, painkillers and alcohol.

In public, Elinor drank very little. She'd occasionally have half a glass of white wine watered down with soda, claiming the ME caused her to suffer adverse effects from the alcohol. Even at home I rarely saw her drink. But she told me she galloped through bottles of spirits, stealthily adding gin to her cups of tea. Certainly, her diaries don't hesitate to record the daily doses of alcohol she'd taken, supposedly to aid sleep or relieve her unspecified pain, but in practice this was a concealed consumption. She once told me she'd 'discovered' a bottle of whiskey hidden in the garage, hinting that it was proof of my dad's out-of-control drinking. But as Dad neither drank spirits nor drank in secret, I can only presume the bottle really belonged to Mum.

It wasn't only alcohol she was guzzling. Having a pharmacist for a father must have been a real boon for someone with Munchausen's, and, even after he died, Elinor writes of her daily self-medicating. She records swallowing tranquillisers, painkillers, anti-inflammatories, Night Nurse, antihistamines, beta blockers, Valium and '*knock out drops*' with increasing regularity from the 1990s. She took them to comfort rather than cure, writing in 1999: '*On painkillers and anti-inflammatories. Don't get rid of the pain but I don't care.*' Perhaps she realised she was addicted – she recorded the phone number for the Council of Involuntary Tranquilliser Addiction in her 1997 diary. Still, she didn't pursue help, and, as her GP seems to have continued to supply her with copious amounts of drugs even after her duodenitis diagnosis, she was able to continue unabated.

Chapter Fifty-Five

Narcissism, Munchausen's and Me

Nanny was a hypochondriac, Grampy a workaholic pharmacist. It's almost too clichéd, since one of the suggested causes of Munchausen's is having parents who were unavailable due to their own illness or a history of working in healthcare. But if that's so, why don't I have Munchausen's?

Mum told me I was likely to inherit the ME and Parkinson's as well as Dad's congenital heart problems, and the diaries jogged my memory. Mum had encouraged me to fake illnesses. Reading the diaries, I recalled a bitter memory, purposefully buried. When I was twelve, I had six weeks off school after having mumps. I remember this time in a few wispy, half-light memories, the emotions embedded rather than words or actions. Even now this recollection is coated thickly in shame, the details hidden in my subconscious, but I remember I wanted to stay home and that it went unsaid that Mum knew I was well enough to go back to school. It was all shrouded in confusion – I can still feel the uncertainty of not knowing if I was ill or if I was making it up. It wasn't clear what was real. I recall the welfare officer visiting, and feeling nervous. I quickly returned to classes after her visit, but my school insisted I went for counselling.

The details of these therapy sessions are hazy. We sat in a small, warm side room with large windows that made me feel on display. You wouldn't see the same set up now; a male counsellor sat before me – a young pre-teen – with my mum sitting in the other uncomfortable chair to my right. It was our second visit, and I shuffled in the seat, letting as few words slip from my lips as possible. Then the tone changed. I don't remember exactly what was said but I know the counsellor turned to Mum and said something about illness. The atmosphere became unbearably heavy. I wanted to get out. I could feel my heart thumping. I wished Mum wasn't there.

We never went back.

'*Not so good this time,*' Elinor wrote of the counselling in her diary, '*Helen decided not to return.*' The responsibility was placed on me, but if you thought your daughter was mentally unwell enough to fake an illness, I doubt you'd let her drop out of therapy after two sessions. No, it was Elinor's decision. '*[Helen] back to school. I was cross,*' she wrote. She was angry at the counsellor. I know, not least because I'm expert in reading Elinor's emotions. I can hear her tone of voice as I read her turn of phrase and I don't need capitals or exclamation marks to know she was seething. But I also know how she felt here, because only when she was furious did Elinor do the housework. Cleaning was martyrdom for her. '*Dusted then collapsed in bed,*' she added. In an archetypal Munchausen's reaction, when challenged about illness, Elinor turned her back on her accuser.

At the time the whole episode scared me, and, though Mum continued to encourage me to take time off school, she writes that I stubbornly insisted I attend. I was so ashamed of this time in my life I hid it in my memory, but, in retrospect, it was a natural inclination. My role model, the only adult inputting into me, was obsessed with illness. There were no aunts or uncles, godparents or family friends, mentors or teachers who had enough access to me to be able to give another world view. Mum was everything. It's more of a surprise that I stood up to her and refused to embrace illness. Why did Elinor become addicted to faking medical problems, while I didn't?

Another suggested cause of Munchausen's and NPD is abuse in childhood. Mum had told me of her difficult childhood, and her diaries gave me the chance to spot her being damaged: a root cause to her mental health disorders, a reason why we had taken different paths.

The diaries start in the 1960s, less than ten years out of rationing, in a Britain physically and financially pock-marked by the war but, contrary to her stories, Elinor writes of growing up in remarkable privilege. With her parents and sister, she took foreign holidays to Belgium and Amsterdam, with overnight stops in London where she visited Selfridges and had a box at the theatre. There are photographs of her in different gowns, long silky gloves and pearls that she wore to balls, and expensive parties were thrown for her birthdays in flamboyant expressions of wealth. In her free time she was constantly shopping, visited the cinema twice a week and went to pop concerts, and her parents showered her with gifts of the latest gadgets and trends.

While I know abuse can hide behind middle-class prosperity, there's no hint that Elinor was even remotely unhappy or scarred by previous mistreatment. Rather than having low self-esteem, she was vain and egotistical, regularly commending herself on her '*long legs*', her '*tiny fingers*' and her ideal figure, while referring to her younger sister as the 'Fat Lump'. Her parents mollycoddled her so much that even into her twenties she refused to take responsibility for herself and she comes across as heartless and spoilt.

As a classic narcissist and a compulsive liar, Elinor's description of her past is entirely untrustworthy. It would only be much later, when I gingerly approached my aunt, that I would find out Elinor lied about her 'difficult' childhood and projected her bad behaviour onto others. It was Elinor's bullying of my aunt, her manipulation and her lies that had split the family.

Instead of outright physical or psychological abuse, it makes more sense that Elinor was over-indulged by parents who were emotionally distant because of their jobs and health issues, which created a perfect storm of conditions. But out of the two sisters, why did it only affect Elinor like this? There must have been something in her DNA to give her the propensity to become a calculating, manipulative narcissist.

Elinor's lies are relentless and the stories she told of her life were exact opposites of what her diaries revealed. Each decade took me by surprise, smashing everything I thought I knew of Elinor's history, but none more so than in my childhood. Her pregnancy journey starts with a jolt. '*Decided I was pregnant so phoned Docs,*' she wrote. Talk about a god-complex; it reads as if I was brought into being by the force of Elinor's will alone. Prior to this omnipotent moment she'd shown no broodiness or interest in children, with only one comment a few years before when she had to babysit for a friend: '*Very off putting.*'

She was characteristically emotionless even at this momentous occasion, describing seeing her scan photos as if watching a nature programme: '*Facinating – awe inspiring*'. Equally, my birth was recorded with cool, plain description. '*Helen didn't cry – gorgeous from start*' is the closest she comes to delight, and I wonder, was I gorgeous because I didn't cry?

At four weeks old I was being held responsible for myself, behaving well for her at the hairdresser's, although later that day: '*Helen misbehaved all afternoon. Didn't get any lunch till 2:45 and not much then.*' What a bad baby I was, preventing my mother from eating her lunch. At ten months old, Elinor writes of me: '*We had put up Christmas decorations but she didn't notice.*' I was born to please her, and, before I was a year old, I was failing.

There are familiar stories from my infanthood, but I find I was only told them in part. I remember the story of my dad rocking me at six weeks old when he accidentally caught my head on a dining room chair. In Elinor's retelling it was presented as a story of my father's negligence, but the diary version is rather different: '*On way [into the hospital] I fell with Helen in my arms – shock and I was treated as hurt both knees. Helen fine thank god. Home.*'

It wouldn't be the last time Elinor highjacked my doctor's appointments, but it's spectacularly cruel for a woman with cut knees to insist on precedence over a six-week-old baby with a head injury. It's farcical to read her entries about her incapacitating grazes over the next few days, while nothing more is said of my bump. Do I need to say I think she fell on purpose?

I was a small, underweight baby, but no concerns were raised even when Elinor ignored medical advice about my allergies. And though reading about this neglect made me shiver, I wasn't overly upset to find it. I removed myself from the situation so I was simply reading a story. Some of the accounts were even funny to me – Elinor's lack of maternal instincts and self-awareness combined with her dry descriptions were ludicrous. It was easy to disconnect, easy to disassociate, and I found myself making excuses for her: she was naive, it was a different time, I wouldn't condemn this if I didn't have children myself.

As I read on though, familiar tales began to take a sinister tone. '*Rang Annette and she asked us to lunch,*' Elinor wrote. I was nineteen months old, and she was 37. '*Nice lunch but Helen didn't eat. Then suddenly Helen had a "funny turn" or mini convulsion!! luckily while I was there. Annette recommended Doc – took Helen home and she slept for an hour and later phoned Doc – he said no problem unless reoccured. Went out in eve to NCT reunion interesting.*'

It's a run of mistakes that, under different circumstances, might have proved fatal: Elinor's lack of concern at her infant having a seizure, the want of initiative to call an ambulance or even a doctor, doing the exact opposite of medical advice and letting me sleep, as well as the GP giving reassurance over the phone without having seen me. I was a baby who needed protecting but, even when events occurred in the sight of others, no one kept me safe.

When Elinor told this story before, it was just a dramatic story. And when I asked why I'd had a seizure, she responded with a shrug – she didn't know and didn't care – because she was at the centre of this anecdote, not me. When I read it now, as a mother myself, the story is altered. I can imagine the heart-stopping horror of watching my beloved baby collapse. I can feel the adrenaline pulsing, my heartbeat tripling, my panicked thoughts tripping over each other. I wouldn't be satisfied to let the situation pass by without seeing a doctor. I wouldn't shrug. It leaves me asking, when does neglect slip into abuse?

Amongst her daily recordings of the weather, her latest shopping exploits, the play dates and coffee mornings, Elinor drops these bombshells in her matter-of-fact indifference. '*To hairdressers,*' she writes. I might baulk at this alone, since having my hair cut was defined as 'me time' when I had a nineteen-month-old toddler; but for Elinor, this is a normal, chore-filled day in November. '*Helen fell down broken drain – oh dear. wet tights, had to fish shoes out of water. Had highlights. Helen had haircut. Got very cold feet but luckily tights damp so walked to car and home to change.*'

Oh dear.

I stare at the words, read them over and over. I see the little girl who tumbles down a broken drain in wintertime, deep enough to soak her tights and lose her shoes. I see the toddler who was cold and wet, frightened and bruised, who, nonetheless, was taken to the hairdresser's to sit for hours while her mother prioritised having her highlights done over changing her daughter's sodden clothes or making sure she's warm and comforted.

These little incidents might raise the concern of friends and acquaintances and strangers, but it's not enough to cause them to intervene. No one would put up with obvious abuse though, would they? It would be easy to spot since abusers look a certain way. A middle-class woman with a perm and glasses, whose appearance and persona tell you she is vulnerable and weak, is immune from suspicion. So, if she wanted to, she could casually walk from neglect into child abuse without fear of reprisal.

I stumble typing the words 'child abuser'. My brain tells me I'm exaggerating. Elinor wasn't a good mother or a particularly nice person, but this is a pronounced turn. I still doubt myself, and I search for excuses. When I read she left her week-old baby in the Moses basket to go to the shops, I tell myself that it was the foolish mistake of a naive first-time mother. Elinor writes that the health visitor scolded her, and, from her account, that was the end of it. Nowadays it would be – or should be – a warning sign, but this was the 1980s and Elinor could easily have played the inexperienced new mum, in need of guidance not chastisement. If the health visitor could brush it off, so should I.

It gets less easy to dismiss. When I was six months old, my parents took me to Bournemouth on our first family holiday. '*Put [Helen] to bed 7:50. Fingers crossed,*' Elinor writes. '*Had meal – good uninterrupted. Sat in bar chatting till 11:30. Walked to beach and back. Hot.*' I can't take the sentences in. I see it, and don't want to see it. I run excuses through my head. I am parenting in a world scarred by the high-profile abduction of a child from a hotel room, hyper aware of the dangers posed. Were 1980s parents more relaxed about leaving their children – their babies – in a room, unattended? Even if they were, there's a difference between leaving your infant alone while you go for dinner and leaving her for at least four hours while you sit in the bar and go for a walk along the beach. My parents repeated that routine every night of the holiday. I see her there, a small baby trapped in her cot, who might have been hungry or wet or lonely, who might have choked unchecked. I weep for her, that tiny, neglected babe.

'*Helen had wind?*' Elinor writes. '*Due to tasting chinese last night? So at 12AM gave her drop of whiskey and she went to sleep.*' It is blunted by time and makes me laugh. My own defence mechanisms refuse to connect myself with that seven-month-old who had been fed Chinese food washed down with whiskey.

'*Gave Helen phenergan in desperation and it worked. 8.10-5.45 without a peep,*' Elinor writes the following June. Phenergan is an antihistamine used to prevent allergy symptoms and motion sickness, but in this case it was used to ensure I slept. Current guidelines state that it is not to be given to children younger than two years old as it can cause severe breathing problems or death in infants. Since there was no connected GP appointment, I suspect Elinor gave her sixteen-month-old baby unprescribed medication. The next day she writes, '*Helen up and sick – sick sick all over me and everything, oh dear. Was it sausage or a bug.*' Or was it that I'd been drugged? Though the names of the drugs change, it isn't the last time this happens.

I imagined abusers would feel remorse or shame, but Elinor makes no attempt to excuse, hide or deny what she has done. Perhaps she thought she was fooling her reader, justifying her abuse by creating a narrative where I was bad and she was the victim. There's no doubt in my mind she wrote the diaries to be read – there are occasional places where she addresses her reader and directs them around the pages – so she may have thought she was manipulating them as masterfully as she did face to face, turning child into parent, baby into aggressor, victim into abuser.

Before I read the diaries, I believed my first memory was of Carys. We were sitting on the stairs in my parents' house in the summer. We were three, peeling melted sweets from the wax paper. But this wasn't my first memory because my timeline was altered by Elinor. According to the diaries, my real first memory was a full year before.

I remember standing on a chair in Annette's house pretending to decorate the wall with a large, blue children's paint brush. I remember falling off and landing on my arm. Mum told me that this happened when I was four.

'*We took [Helen] to hospital,*' she wrote, adding, '*Alan turned up too,*' as if he had coincidentally happened to run into us. '*Helen had x ray – turned out ok but she broke her arm about two months ago – shock horror suspected of baby battering!!! Back to Annette's for late lunch – stayed – Helen fully recovered.*'

Mum embellished this anecdote the more times she told it. She said they'd been interviewed by social services because of the unreported broken arm, though it's unclear whether this really happened. Certainly, nothing came of it, probably because my parents had professional jobs and a nice house and I was clean and dressed well. Though I'd like to think that children suffering hidden abuses like mine aren't brushed under the carpet now, I suspect there still remains a middle-class arrogance that lures us into believing that higher education, prestigious careers and outwardly respectable lives prevent manipulation, deviousness and abuse.

So, how did I break my arm? Mum's verbal version of events was that she'd been putting me in the car a few months earlier. I'd reached back to close the door, and she'd accidentally slammed it shut onto my arm. I'm very careful that I don't repeat this mishap with my children, but, at six, Bailey is just starting to shut the car door himself. I'm not going to argue whether it's realistic for me, at four, to have tried to close a car door though, because I wasn't four. I was two and a half.

When Elinor told me this, it was just another story, but how horrifying it sounds now I am an adult with children of my own. I was a toddler with pudgy little arms, small enough to fit between a pinched finger and thumb. It would have been easy to snap them if Elinor wanted to – if she was in a rage. But who knows if that's what she did; I have no way of finding out.

Though there are no outright episodes of abuse after this, Elinor's tone is threatening. She '*screamed at Helen in frustration*', writes that she '*lost my cool*' and drops in ominous sentences like '*More tears from Helen but shut her up.*' She claimed to be the ideal mother who never smacked her child or raised her voice, but in the diaries she is cruel and out of control, writing '*Smacked Helen's botty that shut her up*' and '*Had to restrain Helen again*'. There are a few occasions where I have unexplained injuries. When I was four she wrote '*Helen fell and cut her labia – very nasty*' and though I was taken to the doctor when Elinor's friend saw my extensive bruises, the GP dismissed them.

The continued neglect is more obvious. I was regularly '*crying with cold*' and even at this young age I was often sent to play alone at the sailing club. Dad was on the water, Mum in the kitchen with her friends, and I remember wandering the waste land behind the club house, weaving between the overgrown dinghies and following trails of small animals. It was boring and lonely. As an adult, I see all the dangers – the cars driving around the grounds haphazardly, the open gate that led to the road, the lack of security or supervision, the endless space to get lost in, the open water. I was a pre-schooler, entirely alone. Unsurprisingly, I read that I was an insecure child who wet the bed, struggled to sleep and barely ate.

Our parents shape our identities, and, in my mother's stories, I was the opposite of the victim I read about in the diaries. Elinor said I was a difficult child who had ruined her life. She said I'd prevented her from having the family she wanted. She said I was always letting her down. She said I was broken. She said my feelings of worthlessness, shame and self-hatred were nothing to do with her. She said I was the problem.

In the diaries, written by my mother's hand, I find a different Helen. A Helen I don't recognise at all. An underweight baby who was left alone for hours in a hotel room and fed takeaway and whiskey. A toddler who was drugged and fractured and bruised, whose needs were ignored even if they were medical emergencies. A neglected and abused young child held responsible for her mother's happiness. All of this happened before I really remember. I have no obvious physical scars and few memories, so these traumatic events are hidden, buried in my subconscious. I've escaped my childhood relatively unscathed, but I'm broken hearted for the damaged little girl I once was: the little girl whose feelings ripple through my life though the stone has long since disappeared beneath the water.

Reading all this sent me into a disorientated fog. I spent months eating biscuits and watching TV in uncharacteristic lethargy. My head felt heavy, overloaded with disconnected thoughts. I couldn't link the Helen I read about with my identity. Nor could I unite the mum I'd loved with Elinor, the child abuser. This wasn't the story I knew – but it is my story.

It's easy not to be angry at Mum. I should be raving, spitting with rage, but it's impossible to summon. I feel the injustice of the situation and I find myself erupting with fury when I think of the doctors and health visitors and friends who saw my abuse and did nothing; but it's an unnatural emotion for me when it comes to Elinor.

As for my dad, he was complicit in my abuse. He should have stood up to Mum. He should have stepped in to protect me. He should have chosen to pour his love and time into me rather than dissolving in drink. He failed me – but rather than finding this upsetting, it's an enormous relief. All this time I thought I'd failed him.

Alan was a dad of the 1980s, a very different creature to Peter. He didn't once change a nappy, and he believed mother knew best. He may well have shrugged off any doubts about Mum's treatment of me because her excuses were so good, her manipulation so convincing. She wielded power over him, most obviously the threat of leaving him, and he loved her. I pity him.

I remember the last time I saw Dad at home before he went to the hospital where he died. He wept as I kissed him goodbye, this strong man I rarely saw cry reduced to violent sobs.

'He's so emotional nowadays,' Mum said with a roll of her eyes, ushering me out of the room as I turned back hopelessly.

Was Dad crying because he knew he was dying and he feared that it was our last encounter? Or was it because he knew his death would abandon me to her? I want the latter to be true, but I see now that Dad never protected me. Deep down I know he would always have chosen Elinor over me.

I might have stayed in that dark place, unable to move beyond the brain-fuddling, contradictory versions of events, if it wasn't for Elinor's therapy journal. In the late 1990s, through her church,

Elinor began having counselling. It started when she fell out with my grandparents. Elinor said that, having become a Christian, her parents and sister cut contact with her. Even when she first told this account, I found it an odd story. My grandparents were highly regarded members of their local church so why would they be upset about their daughter becoming a Christian?

In the winter I was three, the very time that Elinor said her parents disagreed with her because of her new-found faith, there is one line in her diary: '*Then we [Elinor and her parents] had blazing row over Helen, my parenting, Mum and Dad's support or lack of it… Feel depressed, sick of constant criticism.*' Elinor's tale was just another fabrication. She didn't argue with her parents because of her new faith but because they were challenging her abusive parenting. Predictably, when confronted, Elinor dropped the relationship. In her journal Elinor wrote that her mother '*blamed me for being a bad mother*'.

Reading this diary entry, I felt like I was being lifted up, my tiptoes grazing the ground as I rose into the air. I felt my shoulders relax, my headache soften. My grandparents stood up for me. There had been no one else but here, finally, someone had fought for me. I hadn't recalled them incorrectly; the warmth and love and happiness of my memories was real. The photos weren't deceptive – my grandparents really did dote on me. There was love.

During the late 1990s Elinor delighted in having regular one-to-two counselling sessions through her church and recorded her feelings in a notepad. For ninety pages Elinor writes of her difficult childhood, describing feeling like a failure, struggling with self-care, and feeling unloved and unlovable. It starts with petty moaning about sibling inequality, turning into self-congratulatory sentences on her excellent parenting which prevented the ME from affecting my childhood. She writes extensively about her martyrdom as she cared for others to the detriment of herself. I plodded through it, feeling my energy draining, and woke several mornings with my hands clasped around my neck as if Elinor's words were strangling me.

It took all of those ninety pages for it to dawn on me that I wasn't reading Elinor's final truth. Like a magic eye puzzle, as I realised the timing of the journal, my mother's method drew into focus. This wasn't an outpouring of emotion; I was watching Elinor carefully construct her lies. The journal was her cauldron where she mixed projection, falsehoods and half-truths, searching for the perfect concoction to be regurgitated as reality. It was an experiment to find the version that would bring her the most attention and sympathy.

At the time Elinor was writing the journal, when I was in my mid-teens, she records in her diaries that she and I were having lots of 'deep' conversations. It was around the time I had tried to kill myself and I was looking for reassurance from my mum. It was the perfect opportunity for Elinor to feed on my feelings like an emotional vampire, noting them in her journal to use for her own history of abuse. And I wasn't the only person she was doing this to. In her diaries she writes of meeting several people who have had what she refers to as '*difficult lives*'. One person had survived physical, sexual and psychological abuse, and Elinor writes, '*Can't believe how like me [they are].*' She was also obsessed with Oprah and Dr Phil, collecting tragic accounts to amalgamate into her own narrative.

It was only after those ninety pages that Elinor let the truth slip out, adding in some memories that don't fit: '*I've remember that when we moved I was given the bigger room – [my sister] always bore a grudge for that.*' It's a clear memory of being favoured, but that isn't the story Elinor is wanting to tell. '*It's all very strange,*' she writes. '*All the films we went to??? But I had those parties – why did I have the parties. That was me being spoilt. Why didn't [my sister] have parties?*'

These mismatched memories lead Elinor to some self-doubt. '*Am I as innocent as I seem to recall?*' she writes. '*Do I only see what I want to see? Am I so wrapped up in myself I can't see others clearly?*' Here, she's unusually self-aware. '*Was I awful?*' she writes. '*No, passive is the word.'* But even as she tries to fling these truths away, she has to admit that her sister didn't see Elinor as weak and frail as she described herself: *'Sneaky is [my sister's] word.'*

She reaffirms her story of abuse and writes again of the ugly feelings of shame and worthlessness, but then adds: *'I don't think that last paragraph is entirely true. So where does the truth lie?'* Finally, Elinor lets her emotions – her real emotions – run wild. It's the start of a narcissistic rage. No longer the poor victim, she goes on a character assassination, fuming that her mother dared to be depressed, convulsing with shame towards her father and railing against her 'evil' sister who dared to follow the same career path.

Meanwhile, she sees herself as superior, claiming to have *'broken ground'* in her career and *'changed a generation of bank managers'.* *'My mother didn't understand my work,'* she wrote. *'Had no comprehension of my intelligence.'* And she furiously rants about her friends' successes and is incandescent when anyone achieves more than her. Amongst this rage the truth comes spilling out. *'I'm so cross,'* she writes. *'Can't they see how wonderful I am. I'm really special. That's funny because that's what I always believed. I thought Mum was being nice to [my sister] to make up for the fact that she wasn't as nice as me.'*

Narcissists swing between seeing themselves as exceptional and fearing that they're worthless, and Elinor's journal is fascinatingly formulaic. She writes: *'I'm afraid that I'm not good enough. That people will see what I'm really like and turn away.'* But she quickly gets over her self-doubt, returning to fulminating at her long-dead parents, her sister, her friends and even Alan. *'Why didn't you give me the love I needed and deserved,'* she writes. *'You didn't make me feel really special. I felt like an outsider.'* As a cold-blooded narcissist, of course Elinor felt like a stranger in her family, unable to understand her relatives' relationships and feelings. She thought she was superior and doesn't disguise her disgust towards them. *'If you are going to be a professional liar you have to have a good memory,'* she wrote, *'and [they] don't.'*

Through the diaries and her journal Elinor's mask had fallen off magnificently, and it was an incredible relief. I belly laughed when I read those lines, as chilling as they are, because it couldn't be any more glaring. My memories, the diaries and the journal had drawn it all into one cohesive picture. Her vanity, her self-obsession, the Munchausen's, her lack of emotion or care for others, the manipulation, the abuse, the lies the lies the lies – Elinor was a narcissist to the core.

'*We're all special,*' she wrote, '*but I'm really really something special.*'

Chapter Fifty-Six

Out of the Shadows

While I now have a clear view of who my mother was and what she did to me, I still feel like I'll never really know the whole story, never really have a grip on what happened. I have days when nothing feels real, when I don't know who I can trust. I feel like I'm flapping around in an ocean, unable to touch my feet to the floor, treading water while I stay on the long NHS waiting list for a post-traumatic stress disorder referral. Still, the most common reaction I get to what happened is 'How are you so normal?' Honestly, I don't feel normal at all.

My prison all these years has been my perspective, warped by Elinor. There was no one-off event, no easy explanation of this abuse. Rather it was an erosion of truth and trust, grinding me down until my mind was no longer my own and my thoughts and reactions were taken captive. I saw the world through a wall of mirrors and learnt I couldn't trust my point of view, only what Mum told me, even when that changed. Nothing was reliable, and my experiences were a mirage.

Now I'm beginning to really see the world as it is, without distortion, and it scares me. I trusted my mother entirely and completely wrongly, so now my brain runs on hyperdrive, trying to understand what is real, who is authentic and who is good.

I'm tentatively re-establishing relationships my mother sought to destroy – with Judy, with my aunt, with extended family I didn't even know existed. And, most importantly, I'm exploring who I am, chasing dreams of writing and indulging my love of music, established long-term passions I can own without doubt. And beyond the concrete, I daily discover this woman who has been as much of a mystery to me as my mother. A woman with unique beauty, talents and strengths. A woman who is successful, valuable and important. A woman who has survived and will thrive.

Though I've tried to deny it, I also have to accept – reluctantly – that there are many overlaps in my life and my mother's. I can't escape it; we are tied together. Why did I spend years reproaching myself for extending the mumps to stay off school, while Elinor gave no impression of feeling regret for her quarter of a century faking illnesses? I may have affected my education, but Elinor's lies destroyed my childhood, my dad's life and her own. I've carried the shame and failure that Elinor should have felt for too long. Now I understand what it is and why it's there, maybe I can shed it like an old, dried up chrysalis because, despite what she told me, my mother and I are not the same.

It's the middle of July and in one week Bailey turns seven, the summer a glorious, blazing heatwave. The sun shines through our dining-room window, bouncing off a vase of flowers and sending rainbow beams of coloured light across the room.

'What I'd really like is the Lego Death Star,' Bailey says.

Peter and I look across the dinner table at each other and laugh.

'Yeah, I bet you would,' I say.

'Well, definitely Lego,' Bailey says, dipping his pizza crust into some ketchup. He's grown tall, his t-shirts verging into monotone teenage prints, our little boy transforming into a young man.

Blossom picks the pepperoni off her pizza and piles it up on her plate to eat afterwards.

'What else do you want?' she says, flicking back her long hair, sun-bleached strips running through the hazelnut.

'Cherry Coke. A big bottle. Or lime or ginger.' Bailey grins, revealing newly grown big teeth.

Hidden away in a tin is a homemade cake with Darth Vader iced in black, ready for Bailey's *Star Wars* party. Julia says at seven children begin to wrestle with their own identity and independence, forming their own opinions and pulling away from mum a bit more. I've read that emotional abuse by narcissistic parents is often sparked or increased at this point in life too. Elinor's ME began when I was seven.

This is where she and I diverge. Elinor could have chosen a great life, but she didn't. She could have chosen to love, but she didn't. But I will create the best life I can for me and my family. I will love where she did not. I will love wholeheartedly and sincerely even though it terrifies me to be vulnerable.

I watch Peter, Bailey and Blossom planning the party. Without these three I might never have realised the truth or escaped Elinor's grip. The sunlight hits my face and I close my eyes, knowing for certain I've escaped the cave. I continue to stumble, blinded by the brightness, fumbling to make sense of this new world, but I'll never go back. I'm finally in the sunshine.

A Letter from Helen

Thank you so much for choosing to read *My Mother, Munchausen's and Me*. If you enjoyed it and want to discover more inspiring memoirs, just sign up at the following link. Your email address will never be shared, and you can unsubscribe at any time.

www.thread-books.com/sign-up

With the exception of my mother and myself, the names and some identifying features of everyone mentioned in this memoir have been changed to protect their privacy. Although other people who feature in this memoir may have a different recollection of events, this is my truth.

I began writing my memoir for my children, who were too young to understand what had happened with my mother. I didn't want to end up telling them something vague because I'd forgotten the details. And it was just as well I did, because every time I read my memoir through, I'm caught by some detail I've cast to the back of my mind or am overwhelmed by the intensity of the experience. I'm still amazed I came through it.

Growing up in an abusive home messes with your head, and when I was dealing with the ongoing dramas I didn't have the mental space to search for support. But there are organisations that can help if you are going through something similar: not only your doctor or counsellor but social media groups and charities who support people who have been, or are being, abused. I have listed several organisations below (which are mainly based in the UK) for your reference. They have useful information, definitions and advice.

I hope *My Mother, Munchausen's and Me* has touched you, especially if you are going through something similar or suspect someone you know is going through something similar. I hope that my memoir reassures you this isn't a unique experience and nudges you to find support. And I hope that it reminds all of us to treat others with love rather than judgement, especially when we don't understand what they're going through. The kindness I received was essential to my survival.

If you enjoyed reading *My Mother, Munchausen's and Me*, I'd be very grateful if you could write a review. I'd love to hear what you think or about your own experiences around this topic. You can get in touch with me on Facebook, Twitter or at my website helennaylorwriter.com.

Thank you again!
Helen

napac.org.uk
(National Association for People Abused in Childhood)

nspcc.org.uk
(National Society for the Prevention of Cruelty to Children)

samaritans.org (email jo@samaritans.org)

mind.org.uk (email info@mind.org.uk)

blueknot.org.au

counselling-directory.org.uk

helen.naylor.125

HelenNayls

Acknowledgements

I am grateful to everyone at Thread, particularly Claire Bord, who has been an insightful and conscientious editor. It has been a delight to work with her.

Thanks to my agent, Caroline Hardman, and to the team at Hardman Swainson who 'got' my memoir from the first and helped me shape it with astuteness and kindness.

There are so many people who have supported me, not only to bring this book to publication but to get through the ordeal of living through it. I am grateful to my husband and my friends, especially those mentioned in this book, who stood by me during my mother's life and have continued to love and care for me in the aftermath. You were an essential part of my getting through it and writing my memoir and I can't thank you enough.

Thanks also to the inspiring and generous people I met on this journey, in particular Joanne Burn, Graham Caveney, Angela Foxwood and Ibby Maloney for their encouragement, support and advice.

Finally, I am grateful for my two wonderful children. This book is dedicated to you. You are my sunshine.

About the author

Helen Naylor has been writing as a hobby since she was a small girl, but it wasn't until she began a memoir about growing up with a mother who faked illnesses and had narcissistic personality traits that she was encouraged to pursue writing professionally.

Helen lives in Nottingham with her husband, two children and cat and enjoys cycling, playing guitar and drinking good coffee.

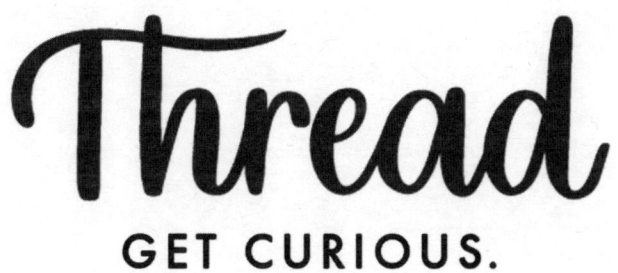

GET CURIOUS.

Join our community

www.thread-books.com/sign-up

for special offers, exclusive content,
competitions and much more!

Follow us for the latest news

@Threadbooks
/Threadbooks
@Threadbooks_
/Threadbooks